TEENS
AND
LOVE
AND
SEX

Charles E. Wittschiebe

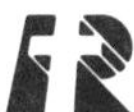

Review and Herald Publishing Association
Washington, D.C. 20012

Copyright © 1982 by
Review and Herald Publishing Association

This book was
Edited by Richard W. Coffen
Designed by Howard Bullard
Cover illustration by Gary Huff

Type set: text, 11-point Palatino
chapter titles, 20-point Palatino

PRINTED IN U.S.A.

Library of Congress Cataloging in Publication Data

Wittschiebe, Charles E.
   Teens and love and sex.
   1. Sex instruction for youth. 2. Sex instruction
for youth—Religious aspects—Christianity.
3. Youth—Sexual behavior. I. Title.
HQ35.W55   1982   306.7'088055   82-12188

ISBN 0-8280-0108-1

Table of Contents

Chapter 1

John and Mary—in Trouble!

John stands more than six feet tall, and his black wavy hair complements his dark complexion. His bulging muscles and agile body make him an outstanding athlete. John is one of the most popular seniors at Black Rock Academy. Maybe it's because of his looks. Or perhaps because he drives a sporty-looking car. Whatever, when most of the girls look at him, they feel all fluttery inside.

Mary, a junior at the same school, serves as art editor of the annual. She has an effervescent personality and participates in most of the school's events. Everybody likes Mary. She has deep-blue eyes and golden hair, and her terrific figure always draws admiring stares from the fellows.

The campus is not especially large, so John and Mary find themselves sharing in a number of school activities. Soon they feel attracted to each other and begin dating. A few weeks later they exchange pictures and pins. Word around Black Rock Academy has it that John and Mary are "practically engaged."

Instead of slowly building a friendship as a basis for courtship, John and Mary bolt into a "deeper" relationship. The physical pull between them grows increasingly stronger. They progress from hand-holding to kissing and hugging then to some pretty heavy petting. Caresses become more and more intimate as John and Mary find that their association revolves around physical attraction.

One night, during a particularly steamy petting session, John passionately blurts out, "Look, Mary. We love each other a lot, right? And we're planning later on to get married. So what do you say? Let's go all the way!"

John's suggestion startles Mary. She had not realized how close to actual intercourse they had come. Her body—stimulated and responsive—wants to give in to John's desire. She loves John and doesn't wish to lose him, but her Christian principles and her parents' training come to the surface. Her eyes mist a bit, and she replies. "John, we can't. I *do* love you, but I want to save that for after marriage." Reluctantly, and perhaps a bit offended, John accepts her gentle refusal.

Over the next few days Mary's emotions clash against each other, and her happy smile no longer spills so readily onto her face. For his part, John is struggling too. During his more reflective moments, he resolves not to press his intentions on Mary. After all, he thinks to himself, he has a moral obligation to protect Mary—even from himself!

Two or three weeks go by, and the constant lovemaking deepens in intensity. The biological stimulation feels so pleasurable that one evening John's good intentions evaporate as he cuddles close to Mary's warm, soft body. Again John suggests intercourse. "After all, Mary," he pleads, "it's the final act of love. You do love me, don't you?"

Again Mary says No to his suggestions, although he notices that her resolve seems just a bit weaker than the first time.

And so, a week later, as they park in a secluded area near the academy, John turns the full force of his persuasion on Mary. He says all the "right" things. He holds and fondles her the way she most enjoys. And he promises unending love for her. Slowly the tension builds. Mary can feel John's passion and realizes that her own responses wildly careen toward the point of no control. And she does love John. And she knows John really loves her.

They have intercourse in the back seat of the car. (We'll talk about intercourse in detail later.) In just a few minutes it is all over. John feels exhilarated, but Mary wrestles with mixed feelings. Sex didn't turn out to be as fantastic as she had thought it would, but she has made John happy. And she does love John.

Time passes. The "final act of love" becomes a regular practice whenever John and Mary go off alone together and park. Mary has lost her virginity, but that's not as important as she used to think it was. She takes great satisfaction in feeling that she now belongs intimately to John. He and she are a part of each other. An uneasy feeling, however, nags her. Shouldn't *she* get more out of sex than she does? Yet she continues to hope that their continuing intimacy will bind John to her more closely and keep her from losing him to someone else.

Mary and John both realize that their activities could lead to pregnancy, but in their minds they "knock on wood" and hope it won't happen to them. They know something about contraception, but neither wants to suggest it. Arranging for protection against pregnancy seems to make the whole relationship more planned, and they want to feel like free spirits, moved only by the force of love. So they just put the whole idea out of their minds. They'll cross that bridge when and if they have to.

Then one evening as they sit in John's car, Mary says softly, "John, I have some bad news to tell you."

"Bad news? What kind of bad news?"

Mary takes a deep breath. "John, I think I'm pregnant."

"Pregnant!" John scuttles away from Mary and turns on the dash lights. "You've got to be kidding. You can't be pregnant!"

"Well, I'm just about certain. I've missed my period, and that's never happened before, even when I've been sick."

John turns off the dash lights. "This is terrible, Mary. You've got to be wrong. Maybe your period is just late or something."

"No, John, I don't think so.

"Well, what are you going to do?"

"Don't you mean 'What are *we* going to do?' "

"Yeah, Mary, sure. That's what I meant. What'll we do now?"

"Well," Mary sighs, "we'll have to tell my folks."

"Oh, man. Your dad'll kill me!"

"Kill you! What do you think he'll do to me? All I've heard from him since I started academy is 'Be careful. Don't lower your standards. Watch out for boys who always want to make love all the time.' "

"Oh, boy, he'll really kill me," John moans. He buries his head in his arms and clutches the steering wheel. The white of his knuckles almost glows in the dark.

"But, John" Mary says, "there's just no way around it now.

We'll have to tell my folks."

They set the time to break the news to Mary's parents. But when the awful day arrives, John's stomach feels terribly queasy and his head throbs. So Mary has to face her folks by herself. She feels that her mother will be more understanding, so waits until she and her mother have the bedroom to themselves.

"Mother, I have some bad news to tell you," Mary begins.

"Oh, Mary, don't tell me you're falling down in your work at school again. Your father and I work hard for your tuition so you can have an education."

"Mother, please wait. It doesn't have anything to do with school. It's about John and me——"

"Now, Mary, you and John aren't breaking up, I hope. After you've managed to land one of the finest boys in the school! I just don't think I could stand to see you lose him."

Mary bursts into tears. She throws herself onto the bed, burying her face in the covers.

"Why, Mary, what is it?" Her mother drops the fresh linen she was carrying and sits next to her daughter. "Come here, darling, and tell me what's wrong."

Between sobs the story comes out. Mary's mother slumps just a bit, and tears brim in her own eyes. "Pregnant? Are you sure, dear? Maybe it's all just a mistake."

"No, Mother. I haven't seen Dr. Richards yet, but I'm sure. I missed my period, and, well, I've noticed other signs, too."

Mary's mother picks up the linen, puts it down, then picks it up again. She rises and moves toward the window and stares blankly out into the yard. "How will we ever tell your father, Mary? I just don't know how we'll ever manage to tell him. You know how he feels about this kind of thing. He'll be furious!"

"Oh, Mom, I can't face Daddy with this! I just can't! Won't you please tell him, please?"

"All right, Mary. I'll try to find a way to tell him. But I think the first thing you and I should do is see Dr. Richards and find out if it's true. There'll be time enough to tell your father later."

A session with the family physician confirms Mary's own diagnosis. She's pregnant. Mary tells John over the phone, but they don't have a chance to talk much about it because John is late for basketball practice. To her surprise, when Mary's father learns what has happened he does not kill her. In fact, he takes the whole situation very calmly. In icy tones he says, "We'll have to consider the alternatives, Mary."

"Alternatives, Daddy? What alternatives?"

"Don't be naive. We'll have to decide what is best to do about this."

"Daddy, I don't understand."

He throws his newspaper down, pushes himself from his recliner, and begins to pace the floor. "We have to make some decisions and we have to make them now. First of all, we have to decide whether or not you're even going to deliver this baby. We may want to arrange an abortion instead."

Abortion! The very sound of the word makes Mary's stomach somersault.

"Or," continues her father coolly, "if you do go full term we will have to decide what to do with the baby."

"Do with it?"

"Mary, don't be stupid! We need to decide whether we adopt it out or keep it and raise it ourselves—or whether you and John get married and keep the child. Decisions, Mary. These are the decisions we've got to make now."

"Well, Daddy, I want to marry John, of course."

"And what makes you so sure that John wants to marry you, my love?" A tinge of sarcasm edges into her father's voice. "He has a bright future: college, business, success. Why are you so sure he'll give all that up and marry you?"

Mary dashes from the room, great sobs tearing from her. How could her father be so unfeeling? Of course John will marry her. After all, John loves her.

But a conference between both families shows that John's parents harbor doubts. They have worked long and hard to get him where he is now, and his prospects seem very bright. Quitting school now would foreclose all possibilities of college and a business career.

And so no definite decision is reached except that Mary will give birth to the baby.

But she does not have a happy pregnancy. Mary has to leave the academy and stay at home when she begins to show. Sue replaces her as art editor of the school annual. She doesn't see

John as often as before, and even when she does, a subtle gulf seems to yawn between them. Mary also notices for the first time how immaturely John often behaves. More and more frequently John calls to say he "can't make it tonight." It begins to dawn on Mary that John's feeling for her was largely physical, and the awareness begins to simmer inside that she has been used rather than loved. John has treated her as a means to an end and not as a desirable end in herself. She feels more like a thing than a person of worth.

By the time Mary has the baby, visits with John have become infrequent. His parents announce plans to send him off to college out West in the fall. They mention something about a wonderful scholarship and a fine work-study opportunity. Mary learns all this from friends who drop in occasionally. John has pretty much dropped out of her life.

She gives birth to a healthy and beautiful baby, and Mary and her mother fall in love with him. He's the first grandson, and Mary occasionally spies her father poking a finger playfully at the little fellow.

Months pass. John has driven to the college out West, and Mary never hears from him except through mutual friends. Her own social needs begin to awaken once more, so she resumes her friendships and activities.

After two years go by, a young man from out of town joins Mary's church. Good-looking, decent, steady, Fred is looking for the right young woman to settle down with. He and Mary meet at a church social, and they find themselves attracted to each other. The friendship blossoms as they enjoy each other's company. Quickly they discover that they have many interests in common.

One night Fred stops by the house to pick up Mary. She's not quite ready, so her parents invite Fred in. He sees a small child playing with blocks in the living room. "Mary, I didn't know you had a kid brother! Where've you been hiding him?"

Mary's face flushes. "Um, he's not my brother, Fred. He's my son."

"Oh, I'm sorry." Now it's Fred's turn to blush a little. "I didn't realize you'd been married, Mary."

The red in Mary's complexion deepens. Her soft voice

reveals a haunting shame. "I wasn't married . . ."

Fred doesn't seem like himself during their date. Frequently he lapses into silence. Mary wishes he'd give her a chance to explain about the baby, but she doesn't know how to bring up the topic again. And it is such a painful thing to talk about. Anguish grows inside her as she senses that Fred will not ask her for a date again. She knows that he is a gentleman and will try to withdraw from the relationship as gracefully as possible, trying to spare her feelings all the while.

And she is right. Fred soon shows up at church functions with someone else. Several months later the entire church excitedly talks about Fred's forthcoming marriage.

That's a pretty gloomy story, isn't it? But unfortunately, this is generally the way it happens. Once in a while the story has a happy ending. "Fred" turns out to be the rare man who has room in his heart to understand and love "Mary" and be a fine father to her son. More times than not, I'm sorry to say, things don't turn out well at all.

How You Came Into the World

Many of you are the firstborn in your families. Now let's imagine how you came into the world.

Your mother and dad met each other, started to date steadily, became engaged, and married. (That was quick, wasn't it?) Then they probably said to each other, "Let's not start a family right away. We need some time to adjust to marriage and to buy some furniture and other things we need."

A year passed.

You mother visited a friend of hers who had just returned from the hospital with a baby girl. While they were chatting Judy asked your mother to hold the baby while she looked for something in the basement. Your mother held the infant close. A warm pleasure crept over her as she played with the tiny hands and cradled the head against her breast. She enjoyed the deep look in the baby's blue eyes, and she fingered her tiny ringlets of hair as she cooed to her. Suddenly your mother craved for an infant of her own. She hadn't realized how much she longed to become a mother.

That evening after supper she said to your dad, "Honey, you

know we agreed to wait two or three years before starting our family. But—would you mind too much if we had our baby earlier?"

"Why, what's gotten into you all of a sudden?"

"Well," she answered, "I went to visit Judy today and had a chance to hold her new little girl. It made me want one of my own."

Then he said, "It would make some changes in our plans, but nothing too important. And if you really feel that way, we can start trying right now. After all," he added with a grin, "you'll have to do practically all of the work!"

So now they made love with the hope that your mother would become pregnant. They had intercourse more often around the time of ovulation—to increase the chance of the sperm's finding a fertile egg in the tube. (All of this will be explained later.)

Mother watched the calendar and her body to see whether her normal menstrual period would come. And, to her disappointment, it did. Another four weeks went by. Again she checked the dates, hoping to pass by her period this time. But no, the usual flow began right on time.

"Won't I ever get pregnant?" she wondered to your dad.

He replied, "Take it easy, honey, we have lots of time. And I don't mind the lovemaking at all."

"Oh, you men!" she blushingly muttered.

The third month neared its end. Mother watched with more eagerness and concern. Suddenly it dawned on her that she was bypassing her period. Not one drop of blood appeared. It seemed too good to believe!

A few days later she told your dad that she believed he would soon be a father. He responded with proud delight and urged her to go to her doctor for a checkup. When she returned, he could tell from her glowing expression that she had guessed correctly.

Right after your mother and dad savored the news together, she called your dad's mother. "Mom, what are you doing?"

"Talking to you, of course, silly. Why?"

"I've got good news for you, Mom. You're going to be a grandmother in August."

"No, you don't mean it! Oh, that's wonderful! We were wondering when you two would get around to presenting us with a grandchild. Are you really sure?"

"Absolutely, Mom. The doctor confirmed it today."

"Oh, I'm so excited . . ."

The same thing happened when your mother called her mother. The two grandmothers-to-be began planning for the grandchild right away. So much sewing and knitting to do, things to buy, visits to arrange. And so much advice to give the mother-to-be about diet, rest, activities, and so on. The expectant grandfathers took it more calmly, of course, but they felt a warm surge of pride at the news. This child would be unusual!

About the sixth month you began to kick. Mother reached over to dad and told him to put his hand on her belly. He felt your movements and asked whether this went on all the time. She said, "No, but quite often."

And he said, "If he keeps on like this, I'll need to have a football ready when he arrives."

Mother laughed and reminded him that the baby could easily be a girl.

Dad gave mother orders that she must not lift anything heavy, that she must avoid falling. She replied that he needn't worry.

As a matter of fact, you were pretty safe. Surrounded by a lot of hydraulic protection, you floated in a liquid-filled uterus. Nothing but a really serious fall or hard collision could endanger you or cause you to arrive too early in the world.*

When the last month approached, dad reminded mother that he wanted her to call him at the first sign of labor. He'd rush right home and take her to the hospital.

Finally the ninth arrived. Dad repeated his request that mother contact him at the first signs of labor pains. Then the last day arrived. She felt the contractions growing more pronounced

---

*By the way, during most of this time your parents still made love. Dad was careful during intercourse and may have occasionally taken the rear position to avoid any pressure on your mother's abdomen. They both enjoyed making love with this variation because it gave him opportunity to caress her clitoris (described later). Certainly the lovemaking didn't bother you. You probably sensed in some dim way the extra pleasure and peace your mother derived from it. It would certainly do nothing to lessen your sense of well-being.

and began to time them. The intervals became shorter and shorter. Mother phoned dad, and he raced home.

Breathless, he dashed into the house and asked whether she was all right. She pointed to her suitcase, and they headed for the hospital. Dad almost ran through a red light and a couple of stop signs. Mother urged him to calm down. They had plenty of time.

Finally she checked into the hospital, and dad stayed with her as long as he could. (In some hospitals the husband can remain near his wife during the whole delivery process.) Later, in the waiting room, he paced back and forth, then plopped into a chair and tried to read a magazine. After what seemed days of waiting, a nurse found him and announced that he had a son (or a daughter).

He replied, "Thanks, nurse, and how's my wife?" (That's the question nurses always enjoy hearing. They like to know that the husband is thinking about his wife and not just the baby.)

The first question your mother asked the doctor after he told her that she had given birth to a son (or daughter) was probably "Is the baby all right, doctor?"

And the doctor happily answered, "Yes, the baby has all the proper equipment. You can take it easy now."

Later dad took the elevator up to the maternity section. He gazed at you through the glass partition of the nursery. You lay near the window, and he looked you over carefully. He thought you had your mother's nose and mouth, but his forehead and chin. The ears could have come from either side of the family. Your hair color more closely resembled his shade than your mother's. Incidentally, you weren't too pretty then, but in his pride and delight your dad didn't notice. (Some men are actually shocked by the physical appearance of a newborn.)

When the day came for mother and you to leave the hospital, dad carefully helped both of you into the car and drove you home. You didn't know what the word *home* meant, of course, but you thrived on the attentions from the soft-handed and soft-voiced person who cuddled you so much. You enjoyed, too, the somewhat less skillful handling of the deeper-voiced person. In your baby way you knew that they loved you, and in your baby way you returned this love.

The Better Way

Well, you have read two different accounts of a baby's arrival in the world. Which seems the better one? You say, "The second one. The one in which they're married." You're right. That's the only way in which a child should ever come—for the good of all concerned.

Every baby is entitled to two parents from the day he is conceived. Notice, I used the word *conceived* and not *born*. And he deserves an honorable entry into this world. Remember, there are no illegitimate children—only illegitimate parents.

These two stories serve as an introduction to the subject of this book—your sexuality.

I have written for both sexes, which means that each of you can read about the opposite sex. After all, there's no reason why you should not be as informed about the other sex as you are about your own. If you marry—and practically all of you expect to do so—you will spend most of your life with someone of the opposite sex. Such a long-term investment of your time and energy makes it wise to get all the information possible so you can increase your chances of having a happy married life. (Or, for that matter, the information could help you to have a happy single life.)

This book primarily addresses teen-agers who are Seventh-day Adventist Christians or who, if not baptized yet, are being reared by Seventh-day Adventist Christian parents.

(Incidentally, I have written a book for parents, too. It is not intended to be a secret guide for them. Instead it's to help them deal comfortably and positively with the subject of sex.)

Chapter 2

To or Not To?—That Is the Question

Unfortunately, the increasing prevalence of pre- and extra-marital sex has become one of the most obvious manifestations of the moral decay in today's world. But we must not allow statistics on actual behavior patterns to establish norms of right and wrong. Surveys can reveal ideas and practices, but they do not provide a safe starting point for making a moral code. God's personality (character) does that. Therefore, Christians do not determine their conduct on the basis of statistical trends. They are leaders in moral living—not followers.

Fornication

The New Testament calls sexual intercourse outside marriage "fornication." The first "General Conference" letter to the churches urged the new Gentile Christians to abstain from fornication (see Acts 15:23-29). In his letters Paul repeatedly warns against sexual immorality. (See 1 Cor. 5:1, 11; 6:13; 7:2; 2 Cor. 12:21; Gal. 5:19; Eph. 5:3; Col. 3:5; 1 Thess. 4:3.) The world of the early Christians didn't frown on such a life style, and in some places religious rituals involved prostitution in honor of the gods and goddesses.

Paul strongly condemns fornication (perhaps with a cult prostitute) in 1 Corinthians 6:18, 19. The believer is a temple of the Holy Spirit. When Christians join their bodies in fornication, they commit sacrilege against the Spirit's temple and against the Lord who owns it, according to Paul's argument. He conveys the idea that fornication is a particularly intimate kind of sin, although we don't know all the implications Paul may have had in mind when he wrote.

Clearly, however, remaining pure is a spiritual requirement for Christians. Perhaps that is why Scripture often speaks of idolatry as adultery, or immorality. But surely the Lord must have had other reasons besides the spiritual for forbidding such conduct. All His commandments spring from His complete knowledge of your nature, including your maleness and femaleness, your needs and desires as sexual creatures. He seeks your maximum happiness and fulfillment. Therefore we can safely assume that He has not forbidden anything merely to show His authority.

I don't believe that the Lord asks you to kill your sex drives. Do you? He doesn't want to mark you off as being not with it, up-tight, or neurotic. He does not aim to form young people into a club of unpleasant fanatics. He does not long for saints with halos on too tight for sensible living.

Therefore you may have heard some people argue that, given human nature and the heavy pressure young people can feel in the area of sex, chastity is an unattainable goal. If a pure life is a practical impossibility, then God must plead guilty to having given you a powerful drive that you cannot control in the way He commands. But God is not unreasonable. The truth is that young adults can abstain from sex before marriage without suffering physical complaints or having their personalities warped.

When you buy a new car, the manufacturer supplies you with an owner's handbook. It explains how you can best care for the vehicle. The human body, with its marvelous sexual organs and amazing capacity for emotional experience, is an incomparably more complex "mechanism." Surely the Creator knows how to give directions for the maximum service and pleasure to be derived from sexual experience.

For the Christian a "Thus saith the Lord" offers sufficient justification for following a particular course of action. Christians are convinced that all God's commands spring from His concern for the happiness and well-being of His creatures. They believe that anything He prohibits thwarts that purpose. But we do not dishonor our Lord when we investigate the possible reasons for His commands. Even if we cannot discover complete answers, what we can learn will reinforce our willingness to comply with His wishes. So let's turn our attention to some of the destructive potentialities in fornication.

Eight Common Rationalizations

People frequently offer numerous rationales for engaging in premarital sex. You have perhaps heard many of these excuses yourself. Most of them suffer from a fatal flaw or two. Let's briefly consider the eight rationales most commonly offered.

1. Sometimes a young man will argue that he needs to pick up some sexual experience before he marries so he can teach his wife all about it. In an earlier generation some fathers would take a son to a favorite prostitute so she could "break him in."

It almost makes sense, doesn't it? Yet the fact is that countless marriages have begun with no experience on the part of either spouse. And these marriages between two virgins have developed into lifelong happy unions. Sex has naturally filled an important place in their marriages.

Being fellow students right from the beginning in the art of lovemaking is by no means an undesirable condition. Think of the many firsts and of the feeling of "just we two" that electrifies all such mutual education and exploration! It's like enjoying a private garden instead of sharing a public park. First experiences can never be repeated, so don't do anything that might detract from that first exciting and beautiful sexual encounter. It should be an event to cherish in the memory.

But chastity doesn't have to imply ignorance in sexual matters. One does not always need to learn by doing. It is important for a young couple prior to marriage to be informed about sexual intercourse, but that information can come secondhand. It can be gained by reading such books as this one.

2. Some couples who are in love may decide that they are already married in the sight of God, so they assume they can freely engage in premarital sex. Or having once succumbed to sexual temptation, they may then argue that the one occasion has made them married in God's sight, so they might as well continue enjoying premarital intercourse.

But they are mistaken. Engaging in sex while not married does not wed two individuals—regardless of their ages and devotion to each other. Since God forbids the relationship, it can hardly become an acceptable form of marriage in His sight.

Because some young ladies tend to equate sexual intercourse with marriage, they may go ahead and marry a young man with whom they have made love. Yet sometimes the man has serious character defects that make him a high risk for marriage and parenthood. A young woman should be alert for such traits. Under such circumstances it would be wisest to end the relationship, even though both parties might temporarily suffer emotionally.

3. Sometimes another argument for premarital sex spins off from the previous excuse. Sexual intercourse, some couples reason, really serves as the true wedding of people who genuinely love each other. "What significance does a piece of paper and a legal ceremony have?" they ask. "Those things are mere forms."

These couples forget that birth certificates, stocks and bonds, passports, deeds, degrees, checks, paper money, et cetera, are also only pieces of paper. But take away their social value and significance, and daily life as we know it would come to a screeching halt, or at least business would jam into a jarring slowdown. Many young women save love letters, wedding announcements, and birth announcements. Are not these only pieces of paper? Of course. But these pieces of paper are all invested with values that we cherish as highly meaningful. They symbolize that which both society and the individual hold dear.

4. Despite what some couples insist, engagement does not give a couple the right to sexual intercourse or conduct that falls just short of this final intimacy. The Christian couple will express affection in ways that they feel measure up to the standards of Christianity. They will avoid any behavior that tends to accent only or chiefly the sensual. They will shun practices that might set a trend for them to "go all the way."

If an engaged couple find themselves participating in activities that drive them closer and closer to intercourse, they may feel it wise to settle on a nearer wedding date. Long engagements can often build up pressures for premarital sex. Quite a few couples fall under the strain of waiting through such a period. The Lord gives power against temptation, of course, but there is no particular merit in enduring long periods that can multiply tensions. At the same time, a couple should take a closer look at their relationship. Is sexual gratification the dominant force impelling them toward marriage?

5. For some couples the resolution to abstain from premarital sex is weakened by the plea that love makes it all right. Such intercourse not only affords a foretaste of the married life to come but also really serves as the true wedding of persons deeply in love with each other—or so these couples reason.

Usually the young man makes the suggestion of sexual intimacy. He often argues that love naturally finds expression in this manner. "If you love me you'll do it," he urges. (Incidentally, many men will do almost anything to get sex, even to claim that they are in love.)

Dr. Sol Gordon states that the most widely used line by fellows is "If you really love me . . ." He suggests that a girl can reply, "If you really love me, you won't put pressure on me." There are many others used to coax girls into sex. Some are fairly common. Others show more "originality."

Real love—mature love—includes self-discipline, self-control, and steady devotion. Young people often engage in fornication on an immature level. The couple can, by habitually indulging in sex in the unreal setting of an affair, become fixated. Fixated means that they become stuck at an immature level of making love. Should they carry this level forward into marriage, it will reveal itself in an inability to sustain the strain of a mature, permanent relationship.

Two of the main ingredients needed in a happy, lasting marriage are character and integrity. Does fornication foster the development of such strengths? Or does it destroy them? Integrity and character do not treat love in a cheap or trivial manner. They do not see it mainly as a physical, sexual relationship. The person with integrity and character sees the physical part of sex as a symbol and fruit of the deeper person-to-person, lover-with-lover relationship. The one-fleshness of intercourse reveals in physical form the one-heart, one-mind, one-spirit union.

Too many of us tend to confuse sex appeal with true love. But sex appeal usually rests heavily on physical looks. Yet if beautiful faces and perfectly shaped bodies were required of both women and men, then few people would get married and few couples would feel sexually satisfied. Sex appeal does not guarantee sexual effectiveness.

Fortunately for us men, women tend to look for those deeper qualities that distinguish a gentleman—with the accent on both parts of the word. And we men should look for those traits that make a young woman a true lady. Leon Salzman puts this all together beautifully by saying: "If I may make a single plea—let us put the person back into sex appeal."

6. In fairness I should mention that the aggressiveness of young women today is rapidly catching up with the aggression of men. One young man (later a suicide at 16) commented on this in his diary. After writing that his dad frequently urged him to protect girls from pressure for sex, he remarked: "I would have liked living in his day. It's like you're not being manly or you can't or you're a queer if you just plain don't want to, or you're waiting, or . . . I don't know what it is . . ."—Beatrice Sparks (ed.), *Jay's Journal.*

These sexually aggressive women seem to feel that it is best to test a permanent relationship before marrying, and this, they assume, includes the sexual aspect. One young lady told me that she would not think of marrying a man she had not previously gone to bed with. She wanted to be certain that the man knew how to "make love." Of course this should include feelings of tenderness, respect, and closeness.

Now, those feelings are desirable—even important—but sexual intercourse does not necessarily prove that they exist. In fact, under these circumstances the sexual relationship itself usually becomes the big deal. Every occasion of intercourse must be an Academy Award performance. Each lover wants to be a star performer in the ability to arouse and respond. Sex becomes so important that it almost separates itself from the personality as a whole—almost like a removable artificial leg. And those nobler virtues of tenderness, respect, and closeness become lost sight of.

Such a focus can easily lead one to undervalue those other elements that make for a genuinely happy marriage. Being too keen on sex can hinder the development of other charms that more likely can guarantee a lasting union.

7. Some men encourage an affair because they want to keep their sexual "muscles" in shape. They seem to regard sex much as a physical education major relates to PE courses. Dr. Paul Popenoe, speaking of this type of man, whom he calls a sexual athlete, once said that he has never known one "who was not completely infantile in his outlook on the world." Hardly an encouragement for a young woman who wants a mature lover.

When a fellow presses hard for sex the girl should ask herself, "Whose needs is he putting first?" If he primarily wishes to satisfy his own needs, does he really love her after all?

Unfortunately, experience indicates that the eager young man who urges premarital intercourse is also most often the one who wants to break up the relationship afterward. He may present the seemingly wise argument that perhaps they both need to look around a bit more before making the final decision to marry. He is trying to say tactfully that he's through and would like to exit without too much of a scene on the part of the young woman. He "forgets" that he told her earlier that they might as well engage in sex because they planned to get married anyway.

8. Some individuals often feel free to ask for sex before marriage as a way to test the partner—of finding out whether or not the other person has a sexual dysfunction (frigidity or impotence). No one has the right to make such a request. Lovers are not entitled to a private undress rehearsal.

Some Adventist husbands who seek the help of a marriage counselor complain about the lack of sexual responsiveness on the part of their wives. Some of them say that they engaged in premarital relations and found the woman to be very ardent. They mention how willingly their wives responded during this period. Now, to these husbands' chagrin, their wives do not seem to be interested. They can't understand why the change has come. If she was *that* good before marriage, they reason, she should be even better after marriage!

I have no way of providing scientific proof, but it seems to me that the problem here could be a delayed guilt reaction. That is, these wives wish they had not so easily surrendered their Christian principles of modesty and purity. They now pay for their sin by unconsciously denying themselves the sexual pleasure of marriage. Or they overcontrol themselves in order to counter-balance their lack of control before. Do you see how this could be possible?

Premarital sex may not prove anything, therefore, about a person's continuing capacity for sexual response. In fact, it may trigger frigidity later on after marriage. Premarital sex can be self-defeating.

Emotional Problems

In addition to the strong attraction that draws two persons together and their rationalizations for engaging in premarital sex, unhealthy motivations can help some individuals slip into such affairs. I'll quickly mention a few of these emotional problems.

1. One young lady became involved with a young man who visited her hometown for a few days. They had engaged in intercourse three times in a one-night date. Later she came to me and said she feared that she was pregnant. Since she indicated that her period was due shortly, I suggested that she wait to see whether she had guessed correctly. A few days later she returned and answered my question by saying, "No, I'm not pregnant." She sounded rather dejected.

"Do I detect a note of disappointment in your voice?" I asked.

"Yes," she said.

"Why is that?"

She paused a while and then said, "Well, I guess I wanted something that would belong to me."

Since I had formerly counseled her mother, I knew a little bit about her emotional background as a child and young girl. I could easily grasp the meaning of her surprising statement and the emotional truthfulness of it. She craved a sense of belonging and wanted to feel needed.

2. Some young people feel uncertain about their masculinity or femininity. So they try to establish their sexual attraction and competence by actually engaging in sex. If their first sexual encounter doesn't meet their expectations—and often that is the case—then they feel even more uncertain of themselves. They become convinced that they are definitely deficient.

3. In some cases the relationship grows out of a gooey kind of sentiment and sick ideas of romance. You find it in songs that say, "I'll love you forever, Baby, till the stars grow cold and the rivers flow backward" or "I'll love you till a day beyond forever, Baby." Life—and love—involves far more than this kind of emotionalism.

4. A few others find in premarital sex a way of dealing with their feelings of loneliness, of being inferior, or of being different. For them physical intimacy cuts down the distance between them and other people—or at least they hope it will. The loved one becomes a symbol of closeness.

Since such relationships often are basically superficial, they bring disillusionment. The pleasure of the act is sharply reduced, and the sense of being desirable as a person—and not just as a sex partner—is diminished.

5. Curiosity and a sense of adventure can bring about some affairs. These affairs rarely last long. The sex partner becomes more of a thing to conquer than a person to relate to. There are much better ways to find adventure than in bed.

6. Escape from an unhappy home motivates some teen-agers to have sex. In their we-two-are-one union, these young people try to heal their hurt feelings and acquire a sense of importance. The young man is king to the young woman, and she is queen to him. Such escape mechanisms rarely solve the problem, however. The sexual organs are too fragile to bear such a heavy responsibility.

7. Sometimes parents are puritanical about sex and have been unreasonably strict in their demands. Under such circumstances their children may seethe with resentment and may take up a sort of careless wildness to show their anger.

Since marriage is one of the traditional pillars of society, these teen-agers make it a point of attack. They complain about the repressions, the hypocrisy, the lack of freedom, and the flatness of life. They try to show their independence by breaking away from the age-old way of establishing families.

8. Not the least of motivations pushing some young people into sexual relationships is the pressure from other teens. Perhaps some of your friends have already told you, "Everybody's doing it." Peer pressure can make you feel that if you

don't do it you're abnormal—or if you don't oblige, someone else will. Such pressure can rest just as heavily on young people as the rules and regulations they're trying to run away from.

9. Underlying much premarital sex is selfishness. Here I want to emphasize the *pre,* not the *marital.* I asked one young man why he did not marry his girlfriend. They were "in love" and had been going to bed together for several months. He put it bluntly by saying, "Why buy the cow when the milk is free?"

When selfishness motivates sexual intercourse, the individual wants to get rather than to give. Yet sexual intercourse should express self-giving. It is the capstone to a loving relationship in which the individual wishes to give himself or herself to the other.

Affairs Create Problems

Many individuals see pre- and extramarital affairs as the solution to many of life's problems. But affairs have their own built-in problems. Persons who engage in such affairs are merely trading one set of problems for another—and most of the time they are the losers for it.

Usually couples must conduct an affair with some secrecy. Often they must resort to outright deception. For many a young woman, at least, a thread of shame runs through it all. She is keenly aware, too, that she does not belong to her sweetheart's family. No matter how intimate the young people may be or for how long, she can never call his mother Mom until after the marriage ceremony. A sense of family and belonging does not grow in an affair, compounding the problem of secrecy and deception.

The more that unmarried people share the intimacy of sex with its overtones of being one, the stronger the woman's feelings of possessiveness become. (Sometimes the man's possessive feelings grow to be just as strong.) Yet always haunting her emotions is the unspoken fear that at any time he may choose to pull out and call the whole thing off. She knows he can say with truth, "Well, we agreed, didn't we, that we would not try to tie each other down—that we'd wait and see whether we were meant for each other?" Most of us expect commitment to accompany sexual relations, but in affairs a personal commitment is usually lacking—at least overt personal commitment.

Probably the great personal intimacy of sex spawns this feeling of possessiveness. A recognized authority in sex education told a class of Vassar freshmen that "there is absolutely no possibility of having a sexual relationship without irrevocably meshing a portion of your two nonphysical selves. Sex is each time such a definitive experience that a part of each of you remains forever a part of the other."—*Redbook*, February, 1964.

Furthermore, should the intimate relationship be broken off, the woman is left with a type of desire that formerly remained asleep. In her sexual experience she has gone "from the cocoon to the butterfly stage." If she has had sex quite often over a period of time, she has grown to accept it as part of being a woman. But with the breakup her life now has the added strain of an awakened desire that she finds difficult to satisfy. She can, of course, find many men who will engage in sex with her, but they will have no intention of marriage. Some women, fortunately, can put this new hunger into a sort of hibernation phase and thus reduce the frustration.

Many young women after a breakup must wrestle with a deep sense of shame and of having been used. Such individuals begin to distrust men and to question their own judgment and instincts in choosing a man.

Professionals who counsel men and women who have had affairs know the pitfalls of pre- and extramarital sex. Wise young men and women will heed the warning flags waved by these experts.

Dr. Joyce Brothers has pointed out that many young ladies are not prepared for the emotional strains of a sexual relationship. Most women are not as "emancipated as they think they are," she writes. Furthermore, the double standard stubbornly survives. Many men prefer a virgin for a wife, she observes, and some men feel that a nonvirgin wife will more likely have an affair after marriage. Dr. Brothers sums up her discussion by saying that "people often ask of sex more than it can possibly give" (*Good Housekeeping*, June, 1969).

Dr. John E. Cavanagh, a Catholic psychiatrist, says that "sex is only incidental to premarital happiness, and sex before marriage leads more to unhappiness than it does to happiness. In fact, I believe quite honestly it can be said that sex causes much more misery than it produces pleasure."—*Medical Aspects of Human Sexuality*, May, 1973.

No one can charge Dr. David Reuben with being unenthusiastic about sex. Yet he states that "sexual performance BEFORE marriage is absolutely no indication of sexual performance AFTER marriage" (*McCalls*, February, 1971).

Experts generally agree that marriage and just living together are different. Living together before marriage, they point out, can prove only one thing: that two people can live together happily before marriage. (You may have to read that two or three times to get the point.)

I like the way Sydney J. Harris in his column in the San Francisco *Examiner* put it: "It is simply that firing blanks is not the same as exchanging bullets. . . . No informal living arrangement, even for years, can simulate the stresses and tensions and responsibilities of the conjugal state."

In a sexual survey reported in *Medical Aspects of Human Sexuality* (May, 1979) five hundred psychiatrists were asked: "In what manner does sexual experience usually affect a teen-ager's personality?" Six out of ten said that it "increases confusion or conflict."

Perhaps now it is easier for you to understand that when God forbids fornication, He is not being arbitrary. As a loving and concerned Father, He wishes to protect you from any behavior patterns that could in the long run destroy your physical, emotional, and spiritual health. He wants you to achieve true manhood and womanhood. He looks forward to your attaining the richest possible experience in marriage.

Chapter 3

Illegitimate Parenthood

Have you read the statistics on teen-age pregnancy? If you haven't, you're in for quite a shock. According to a report in *Newsweek* (Sept. 1, 1980), nearly half of the nation's teen-age young women between 15 and 19 years of age have engaged in premarital sex. And each year one million of these teen-age young people will learn they are pregnant. That's 10 percent of the U.S. female teen population.

Contraception

You can hardly live in this world without knowing that you can use birth control methods to prevent the conception of a baby. And surely you'll agree that the production of an unwanted child is one of the cruelest acts of immorality. No baby should come into the world because of a couple's impulsive mood or because two people carelessly neglected using a contraceptive method. (When you marry, you will certainly plan to use some method that will allow you to control the number and spacing of your children. There is a reasonably wide choice open to you and your future mate.)

I have written this book with the assumption that as a Christian you will not engage in sex before marriage. Therefore you will not need detailed information about contraception. However, if you have not placed your sexuality under the Lord's control, you ought to take responsible precautions to prevent the conception of a baby. You may have to face the painful choices of having an abortion, putting the baby up for adoption, of being a single parent, or of entering a forced marriage. In any case, remember the earlier comment on page 15: There are really

28

no illegitimate babies, only illegitimate parents.

Keep in mind, too, that babies can make big changes in vocational and educational plans. The arrival of a baby can strongly affect the emotional growth, for good or bad, of both persons involved—whether the baby is allowed to live or not. (Notice the grimness of that last statement.)

The responsibility for contraception in most premarital affairs usually rests with the young woman. Yet if she prepares herself against conception or comes equipped to meet the possibility of intercourse, she appears to be too aware of the sexual relationship and too "practical" for spontaneous intimacy.

The young man may not want to appear to be expert in the use of a contraceptive (and often he is not) for fear that the young woman will wonder where he picked up his experience. Most men prefer to think of sexual intercourse as the natural consequence of a growing buildup of desire.

In short, neither partner wants to plan on getting carried away. The high point of sexual intercourse is supposed to sneak up on them, they think.

As you know from talking with your friends and from reading about the subject, there are different levels of knowledge about contraception. Many teen-agers still know very little about sex. Although ignorance is only one reason for not using some form of contraceptive protection, it plays a part in the dangerous gambling that teen-agers participate in when they indulge in sexual intercourse.

Some young people feel that pregnancy will most likely not occur if they do not have sex on a regular basis or if they confine their intimacy only to the safe period. ("Safe" in this case depends on their arithmetic and their knowledge of the menstrual process.)

Still others assume that the use of a contraceptive will cut down on the pleasure and thrill of the sex act itself.

Quite possibly some teens may have an unconscious need to be punished for their wrong conduct. Pregnancy can then serve as that punishment. The baby can be a sort of atonement for indulging. One wonders, however, who would suffer more in such a situation—the parent or the innocent infant?

Many young women feel that the pill provides the most certain form of protection. And it does if the young lady commits herself to a constant and unfailing schedule of pill-taking. To get on such a program seems to imply a commitment to the idea that sex will be an expected part of the date. The use of an intrauterine device conveys the same impression. Most other methods of contraception are less convenient and more likely to break the rhythm of the lovemaking, particularly when it occurs on "unexpected" occasions.

A number of young people practice as intimate sex as possible without actually engaging in intercourse. We call this "technical virginity." These lovers engage in passion-arousing caresses that lead to orgasm and ejaculation apart from actual intercourse. This can include manual stimulation, oral stimulation, oral sex, anal sex, and between-the-thighs intercourse.

The Christian, however, does not see how far he can go in breaking the spirit of the seventh commandment and yet absolve himself by saying he has not been guilty of immorality because he has not entered the woman's vagina. These practices are to the seventh commandment what beating a man half to death is to the sixth commandment!

Practicing technical virginity with between-the-thighs intercourse not only is immoral but also is a poor form of contraception. In certain cases fertilization does occur. Sperm deposited on the opening of the vagina have found their way to the waiting ovum.

A young wife with whom I was acquainted had this happen to her. Before their marriage she and her fiancé (now her husband) wanted to get as close as possible to the real thing. They settled for intercourse between her thighs. Soon her periods stopped, and she began to feel sick every morning. Since, by her own story, pregnancy could not be a possibility, her doctor did not at once order a pregnancy test. However, after eliminating other possible causes for her symptoms, he took that step. To the consternation of the young woman and her fiancé the test indicated that she was pregnant.

Perhaps the most fitting conclusion to this section is Dear Abby's pithy remark that the perfect oral contraceptive is the word *NO*.

Reasons other than refusing to use contraceptives may also lie beneath the surface of a pregnancy. A young woman, for example, may want to prove to everybody that she is feminine. She may wish to "get even" with her overly strict parents. She may want to keep up with a relative or friend who has just discovered that she is pregnant. She may feel she needs to prove that she is grown up (forgetting that children can have children). She may seek a way to get out of school. Or perhaps she feels a deep inner need for someone to love who will be all her own.

Possibly the young lady may want to tie the man to her by a strong bond of sharing—50 percent of a child can be a pretty heavy commitment, especially if the man has any decent instincts and any sense of responsibility. However, in this connection it is only fair to mention that the majority of today's college women who live with partners "without benefit of clergy" do not expect marriage as the next step in the relationship.

Sometimes the young man may feel that he can demonstrate his manhood by engaging in intercourse and making his partner pregnant.

Both partners may have an unrecognized undercurrent of desire to bring on a pregnancy because they have set their wedding date too far into the future. A baby on the way can provide an almost unbeatable argument for bringing things to a head and for moving up the time for the wedding ceremony.

Pregnancy Involves More People Than the Couple

An impending pregnancy for an unmarried couple has a decided ripple effect. The young people involved really put their parents in a terribly distressing dilemma. Do they disown their children and let them lie in the bed they have made? Do they wash their hands of any responsibility? Or do they rally round to support their offspring (including financial support) and help them make the best of an unplanned birth that shatters all the hopes they had for a more normal future in terms of education, time of marriage, and starting a family? (Incidentally, I am impressed from my experience over the years by the decent and kind way most parents react to becoming unexpected grandparents.)

The area of responsibility gets even wider. Not only the pregnant girl and her parents (natural or adoptive) but the larger family—the church and society—becomes involved. The people in the community may have to pay taxes earmarked for aid to dependent children.

If the young woman decides to have an abortion she may find herself besieged with guilt feelings. Although unmarried women find it easier to obtain an abortion today than a few years ago, large sectors of society continue to frown on abortions. So the burden of guilt can be doubly hard to bear.

Adoption in such pregnancy situations may appear to be the better plan for both mother and child. Of course, she has the nine months of carrying the baby. And in many cases a bond begins to grow between the unborn child and the mother-to-be. Breaking that tie and giving up the "fruit" of her body to perfect strangers is for many women a wrenching and tearing experience. For this reason many mothers, when they have given birth to the baby, do not look at it or hold the infant. This way they can avoid becoming even more emotionally attached to it.

The baby, however, goes to a home hungrily awaiting the child. Competent persons have usually carefully checked out the prospective parents. Their motives for wanting a baby must be healthy and their fitness for parenthood evident to the investigating authorities. In such a family the child will very quickly seem to have been born to them. They will even imagine physical resemblances. There will be love and concern, a home and a father, and grandparents, cousins, aunts, and uncles. (Some "adoptive" grandparents have to come around to the idea of having a grandchild that way.) The adoptive parents will need wisdom and tact and unselfish love so that they can convey to the child the delicate shadings of adoption. As you can guess, it takes more mature love to be an adoptive parent than a natural one.

It is not at all rare for a pregnant teen-ager to find that her lover has lost interest in their relationship. Selfishly and gracelessly he leaves her to work her way out of the situation alone.

Sometimes single parenthood is the best option open to the

young mother. However, to be the unmarried mother of a child is not an easy lot in our society. In practically every case the mother must work to support herself and the child. If she continues living with or near her parents, the problem of a baby sitter may be solved. But it is one thing to visit one's grandchild occasionally, and another to have the full care of him or her for forty or more hours a week. Still, if the grandmother is in her early 40s, she may derive some pleasant excitement from caring for a new baby. It can make her feel as if she were having a menopausal child.

If the grandmother does not live close enough to care for the baby, an older married sister may live nearby. Failing such help, the mother will find it difficult to get the same quality of care and concern that someone within the family would provide. When one does find a suitable person, the cost can take a large bite out of the weekly paycheck.

Under such an arrangement the mother keeps the baby, but she can't share many of the vital daytime hours with her child. As the youngster grows older the mother becomes increasingly aware of the child's need for two parents. She senses more and more that she cannot possibly give the physical and emotional nurturing a father can provide. Of course, the grandfather and uncles (if the mother has any older brothers) can to some degree substitute for the missing father. Even at best, however, the child deserves more than these relationships provide.

As the baby grows older the difference in the homelife begins to dawn on him or her. The child will feel odd with only one parent. The later knowledge that he or she was born out of wedlock can trouble the maturing youngster increasingly.

The Had-to Marriage

Studies have shown that some of the involved young men stand willing to help in the expense of the child's delivery and are ready to marry the expectant mother.

When a women goes through nine months of producing a baby and through the wearing hours of birth—with all the physical and emotional stresses involved—she deserves to have a man standing by who loves her, is committed to her in marriage, and happily shoulders his share of the responsibility for the child. She should have the pleasure of introducing the baby to the man not only who is the natural father but who has also placed himself on record for all to know that the child is his. No woman should have to go through pregnancy and childbirth by herself. It can be a painfully lonesome road.

Expenses for the young couple can be a heavy, if not stunning, problem. Without doubt, by their cutting corners and by borrowing some things, costs can be reduced. But the heavy expenses that remain can come as an unpleasant introduction to the economics of marriage and parenthood—and one from which some couples never recover. In many cases the couple must jettison their educational and vocational plans and cope with a lifelong disappointment.

If her boyfriend marries her when she's pregnant, the girl may wonder a bit later whether her pregnancy pressured him into a proposal. She has heard through the years of shotgun marriages and may feel that hers falls into that category. Naturally she wants to think that he would have married her no matter what happened, simply and only because he loved her. But under the circumstances there is no final way to prove that, except by his continuing love and faithfulness in the marriage.

Whatever the reason for marrying, statistics indicate that young people who marry in their teens are three times as likely to break up their marriages by divorce as couples who wait until they have matured more before getting married.

To be fair I should mention that some forced marriages do turn out well. Some unions are stable and happy, and both husband and wife seem to accept their responsibilities without self-pity or bitterness. Perhaps the degree of emotional maturity that both partners exhibit has a lot to do with these success stories.

Future children within the marriage may also suffer under some fallout from the parents' experience. The individual parent can repent and be forgiven and mature into a deep spiritual experience. But sometimes a hidden, almost unrealized, sense of guilt works against the self-confidence and self-respect needed for parents to impart the right kind of sex education to their children.

One mother asked, "How do you advise your daughter

against premarital sex when you had it before you married your husband (but now wish you hadn't)?" An answer to this question is that a frank discussion of the past may be the most powerful argument of all.

On the other hand, a revulsion against one's past sinful conduct may bring about a too-severe strictness in sex training. One's effort to keep a daughter, for example, from making the same mistake as her mother may lead to overprotectiveness and unhealthy shielding from the normal temptations of young people.

Some investigations indicate that experience in premarital intercourse seems to make it more likely that an individual will engage in affairs during marriage. But a lack of trust within a marriage can wreak havoc with the relationship. Mutual trust and commitment and love can serve as the glue to keep a marriage intact.

When the Affair Breaks Up

If a teen-age affair ends without marriage, as many do, then the young people have another problem to face. If the woman later finds the man of her choice, does she tell him she is not a virgin? Or what about the young man? If he has had previous sexual experience, should he confess to his fiancée?

Let's deal with the first question first. If the young man involved is a virgin himself and has always dreamed of having a virgin for his wife, the young woman ought to explain her situation, and the relationship probably ought to be ended. (It seems as though somewhere along the line as their feelings for each other grow that the young woman would have detected this expectation. After all, women are quite intuitive about such things.) To hope later for a complete adjustment on his part to the disturbing revelation is, in many cases, expecting too much. A marriage in which the past hangs over the two like a dark cloud always has the potential for large amounts of tension.

The situation is not completely hopeless, of course. If he would be willing to seek professional guidance, a counselor could probably help him get his feelings up to a level where he could deal with them comfortably. But if he cannot resolve his feelings of jealousy and distrust, then the couple are much better off to go their separate ways—as painful as that may be.

The second question refers to the young lady's feelings. If the young man has not preserved his purity and if she can't forgive and forget, then the couple should most likely break up. However, I have found that generally a woman will forgive a man for his past misconduct particularly if she is convinced that he considers these past affairs as steppingstones to the great and permanent love of his life—herself.

A man who has lived a wild life or made one or two missteps before conversion and who then finds a chaste young lady who loves and marries him often considers himself to be one of the most fortunate men in the world. He wonders why his wife cares so much for him despite his past. She inspires in him a kind of reverence.

Even though a couple may have to go through the trauma of ending a relationship because one of the parties finds it impossible to forgive and forget, a person does not need to wrestle with guilt for the rest of his or her life. The violation of the seventh commandment is serious, but it is not the unpardonable sin. Perhaps one's lover cannot forgive, but God can. He can cleanse the repentant sinner from a past life of impurity. His love turns away from no confessing sinner.

Chapter 4

Chaste or Chased? It's Up to You

It seems almost unnecessary to mention that sexual attraction ought to be present in courtship, as well as in marrige. To date or marry simply because the other person has money or because one's friends are marrying or whatever other motivations might impel you means taking a great risk. Biological attraction should furnish the electricity for the relationship, but it should not be allowed to become so overpowering that it short-circuits the entire relationship.

Through courtship, engagement, and marriage you can build the most intimate man-woman relationship on the principles of 1 Corinthians 13, the love chapter. In true love each of you will grow as a person and as man or woman. And there are ways by which you can recognize true love. You feel more alive when you are with each other. Each brings out the best in the other. Both of you are proud of each other. You feel especially blessed in finding each other.

How to Keep It Proper but Fun

There are also ways to keep sexual urges from dominating the courtship and ruining a beautiful relationship.

A young couple should examine their inner workings. Are motives other than love pushing them into the relationship? Is one of the parties running away from something as much as running into something?

A Christian will select friends—and dates—carefully. Don't pick a date merely because other people don't like him or her or because that person looks like a motherless child or because the individual needs to be saved. Dating is not a form of evangelism.

You must not let pity or Christian concern or a desire to fight for the underdog involve you in an emotional relationship that could lead to a disastrous marriage.

Conversion and reformation should be in the past before you take any chances that possibly could unite your life with someone who has traveled the wrong road. This does not, of course, rule out normal and helpful social relations, particularly within the protection of the larger church family. You don't want to assist the devil in setting up temptations by your association with persons who are wild or unprincipled or "lovers of pleasures more than lovers of God." You will also want to stay away from those places that such individuals frequent.

Christian couples avoid late hours, lonely places, and suggestive moving pictures or shows (including those on TV). They do not want sex to become the central drive in their relationship. Therefore they avoid sexually stimulating activities and places. They refrain from any intimate caresses, being guided by the principle of modesty. To many of you this may read like something out of a Victorian guide to conduct—far removed from life today. But let me assure you that there are Christian young people who do maintain these standards.

For the same reason you will select carefully the kind of music you allow yourself to enjoy. Music can be, and often is, a part of the getting-to-know-you and the courtship stages. You live in a period when for the first time a whole new type of music is being composed for young people—by young people.

This music often deals frankly with sex and sometimes with such practices as masturbation and oral sex. Sometimes the references are quite obvious. Other music ranges from the obvious to the completely explicit in terms of intercourse. This can occur both in the words and in the gestures that accompany the song. The musician, for example, frequently uses his instrument as a visual aid in creating the fantasy of intercourse.

As Seventh-day Adventists you will abstain, of course, from drugs and drinking. These often go hand in hand with immoral behavior. Further, you will want to include the milder drugs like coffee and tea on your "not used" list. You want to keep your bodies in peak condition so you can give your children a good start in life. Some recent tests suggest that caffeine may cause birth defects.

Health-conscious young people also avoid junk foods and drinks. They use good judgment in their use of time for work, rest, study, and recreation.

A strong physical body is an unequaled basis for a healthy mental, emotional, and spiritual life. Since you have heard this from childhood days, you may take it for granted without making it a definite part of your life.

It may seem that premarital sex has become so common that the person who tries to maintain a code of no fornication appears sick or odd. One should never forget that true Christians are always a small minority in the world and, unfortunately, sometimes only a slightly larger minority in the church.

Right from the beginning of a relationship a young woman can make her standards of sexual conduct evident. She even has the right to make these a condition of future dates. She can defend her position without having to feel defensive or neurotic. Just because she asserts her right to remain a virgin until marriage doesn't necessarily mean that she's a prude or a misplaced Victorian.

Furthermore, a young lady does not have to be extremely kind in turning down an offer to have sex. An invitation to engage in premarital sex is basically an insult to a Christian young woman. It deserves an indignant and sharp refusal.

Note Mrs. White's comment on this kind of conduct: "If a young girl just entering her teens is accosted with familiarity by a boy of her own age, or older, she should be taught to so resent this that no such advances will ever be repeated."—*Testimonies,* vol. 2, p. 482.

If a young woman sees the possibility of passes on future dates and wants to handle the situation with appropriate humor, she might send the young man a jesters card (40572C), available in many card stores. The cover says, "Before we go any further, there's something you should know about me." On the inside page are these words: "I'm NOT going any further!!"

A Christian young man will want his love to include respect for his date as a person, respect for her Christian standards, and a self-control that is not always teetering on the edge of breaking down. Some young men will take offense when young ladies refuse their proposition and will quickly withdraw. But a Christian will decide that such a fine young lady is worth waiting for.

Conduct your courtship on an honest and open basis. Make both pairs of parents aware early of the more serious intentions both of you have. Respect them for any counsel they give and for the protection they can furnish for your good name.

Give your parents progress reports on the relationship. Provide them with the chance to size up the fitness of the prospective fiancé or fiancée for the responsibilities of marriage and parenthood. You want your parents to welcome your lover as a prospective part of the family. You hope that your brothers and sisters feel that you are about to make a delightful addition to their ranks. Each of you will come to consider the other's family as your own—so much so that later the in-law ending in introduction seems unnatural. Incidentally, Mrs. White referred to her daughters-in-law as daughters.

(Now and then a parent may neurotically try to hold on to a child. For example, dear mom may want to keep you always with her. She may even resort to emotional blackmail by making you think she's going to become dangerously sick if you leave her. If you have such a parent [such parents are not common, fortunately], you will have to preserve your own right to independence. A counselor can help you make the break with as little shock and distress as possible.)

Don't rush to become engaged. A high proportion of first engagements among college-age young people are broken. The engagement should put the seal on a friendship and courtship that has taken into account all the factors necessary for a good marriage.

Looking Forward to Marriage

So take a good look at all the possible motivations you have for marrying. If you have any hesitation or any second thoughts, confer with a counselor whom you trust. Search before marriage is always better than search later—to avoid making a lifelong mistake.

As part of your wedding preparation I hope you consult a

minister for a few periods of counseling. Do this as far ahead of the wedding date as possible. (In some cases the interviews may bring to light unreadiness for marriage or the inadvisability of this particular one.) Or you may choose to visit with a professional counselor. If so, you will want to give your pastor permission to communicate with him or her.

During your first year of married life it would be smart for you to return to the counselor for an "oil check." Since the first year or two require both of you to make many adjustments, a checkup on progress can prove helpful. Of course, in time and by experience couples usually work their way through these adjustments, but a follow-up visit with your counselor can often reduce the amount of strain and hurt produced even in a very compatible union.

Nowadays it is also necessary to recognize the influence of divorce when you choose a mate. The tendency to divorce runs in families. Prof. J. T. Landis back in the fifties reported some interesting findings. If neither pair of grandparents had been involved in divorce, there was one divorce in 6.8 marriages among the grandchildren. If one pair of grandparents had this misfortune, the ratio rose to one divorce in 4.2 marriages. If both grandparental families resorted to this drastic method of ending a marriage, the ratio went up to one divorce in 2.6 marriages.

Now, a history of divorce in the family does not cause an indelible taint. But it does mean that extra care should be exerted in picking a mate from such a background.

Some children from such families are even better prospects for a good marriage. They have suffered the consequences of divorce, and they have made up their minds that they will *never* allow divorce to ruin their home.

As you move on, in your later teen years, to marriage, you can greatly reduce the risk of divorce by wise Christian behavior.

In looking forward to marriage some young people, especially the brides-to-be, anticipate doing everything together always. The two-become-one concept is pushed to an unreasonable level. Even in a happy marriage each spouse may at times wish to be alone. (I am not thinking of a separation of weeks and months.) It is a form of strength—and often a need—to be able to enjoy privacy and to move about in one's own living space.

Togetherness can become cloying and smothering—especially if it arises out of an inability to feel secure when alone.

Very likely most of you will feel obliged, after marriage, to work outside the home. Arrange to have the job program interfere as little as possible with the rhythm and closeness of your marriage. Avoid working on different shifts—or pretty soon you will have the feeling that you are making love in a revolving door.

In today's world a young lady has to prepare not only for a home but also for a vocation. Even if she doesn't plan to work after marriage, she needs to keep in mind the possibility of future circumstances that might make it necessary for her to return to the job market.

I don't like to tell you prospective wives this, but if you do work you will probably carry a larger share of the family responsibilities than will your husband. Very few men help their working wives with 50 percent of the household tasks and the child care that you would expect in a fair division of labor. When you select your husband, find out how willing he would be to pull in equal harness with you. One way to judge how he will act later is to observe how his father treats his mother if she works, or how he himself treats his working mother. Of course, if the young man feels that his father is not fair with his mother he may intend to do just the opposite when he marries. Observation and tactful questioning can furnish a lot of useful information.

Some men want to go from the mothering of a mother to the mothering of a wife without doing much more in their new homes than they did as a teen-ager in their premarriage homes. No man is so wonderful to have that you need to baby him or spoil him to keep him around. You are better off single. Ask any overworked wife and mother!

Marriage is an exciting prospect for young adults. It is one of God's finest gifts to His children. But remember this during your years of courtship: Marriage is not a destination; it is a journey. During the next few years read frequently the comments on courtship and marriage found in *Messages to Young People* and *The Adventist Home.* You will doubtless be surprised at Mrs. White's timely and sensible advice.

Chapter 5

For the Fellows

Anatomy

Penis—You fellows are more aware of your sex organs than girls are of theirs. After all, you can readily see your penis and scrotum. (A young woman's breasts are highly noticeable, of course, but they are not "mainline" sex organs.)

Some of you worry that your penis is too small. When you are in the shower room with other fellows, you make comparisons (without letting them know you're doing it). Actually, rarely does a man have a penis that is too small. The length of the penis "at rest" is two to four inches and when erect, four to eight inches. (From here on all sizes, weights, and shapes are only approximate.) When you look at your own penis from above, it appears smaller than it does to others—or to you if you look at yourself in a mirror. And, good news, smaller penises when erect increase proportionately more in size than do larger ones. So it's not so much where you begin as where you end!

Of course, size is not the real worry. You really fear that you won't be as good at sex as the next fellow. You can forget about this fear because being good at sex doesn't depend on the size of one's penis. A woman's vagina is most stimulated at the entrance and near the opening. She has little sensation farther in, except of fullness and gripping—and friction caused by thrusting.

A second point. Your future wife will love you for the man you are and not for the size of your penis. She will be more concerned with the quality of your lovemaking. True lovemaking, even in intercourse, depends on trust, sensitive sharing,

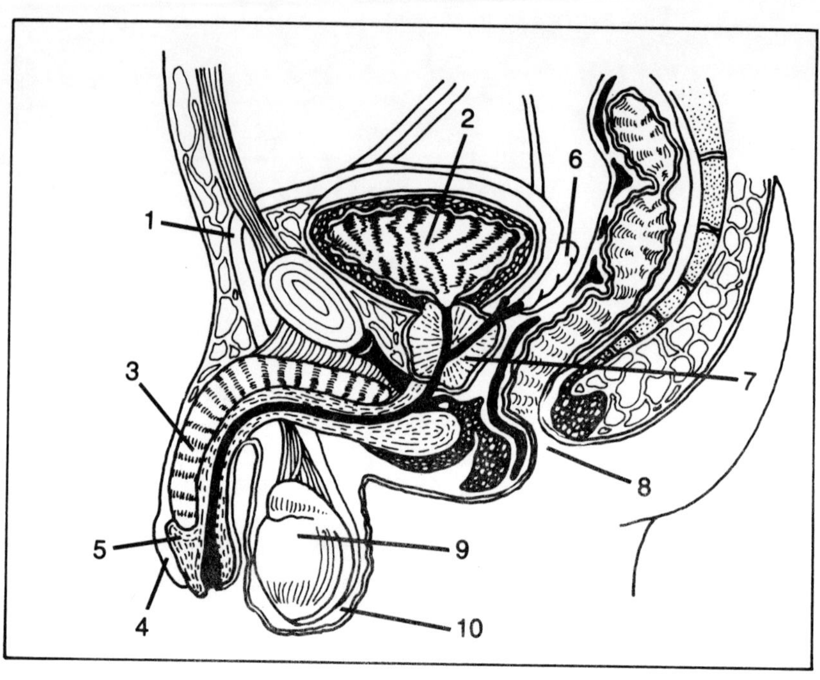

1 spermatic duct

2 bladder

3 penis

4 foreskin

5 glans penis

6 seminal vesicle

7 prostate gland

8 anus

9 testicle

10 scrotum

The male reproductive organs

deep communion, and a feeling of intimacy shared by no one else in the world.

To sum it up, your success in sex as a husband will depend not on the size of your penis, but on the size of your heart—the emotional one, that is.

By the way, exercise does not increase the size of the penis. Encouraging erections won't make it any larger. It isn't a muscle.

Although the organ is quite small when not reacting to sexual excitement, during an erection it will extend to about six inches in the average man. An erect penis looks somewhat like a mushroom with a small head and thick stem. The head of the penis is extremely sensitive, because it contains a mass of nerve endings.

Probably four out of five male infants in the United States are circumcized shortly after birth. In this operation the physician removes the prepuce or foreskin—a fold of skin covering the head of the penis. Circumcision leaves the head of the penis exposed. Some people today argue for circumcision because it aids in keeping the penis clean of smegma (a cheese-like substance that accumulates under the foreskin), and because some think it helps protect a man's wife from contracting cancer of the cervix. Others offer what they consider to be strong arguments against it.

These points, however, are hardly likely to account for the Lord's choice of this rite as a sign of dedication for Abraham and his descendants. In those days the woman who married such a man shared in his symbolic dedication. And since the penis conveys the sperm in the act of intercourse and thus has the high honor of being the means by which man shares, at the creature level, in the creative power of his Maker, circumcision most likely symbolized commitment to God at the very deepest levels.

Scrotum—The pouch under your penis is called the scrotum. If you've ever played as a catcher without wearing a protector or an aluminum cup and had a ball whiz across home plate and graze you as it passed between your legs, you know how sensitive this area is. Or if you had a rope get caught in your crotch or if you slid off onto the bar on your bike. Men unconsciously tend to protect this part of the body. Stewart Alsop, the famous journalist, was on a plane flying over enemy territory. Antiaircraft shells exploded around the plane, and it bucked wildly. As he glanced around the cabin he noticed that every man had his hands crossed over his midsection.

The scrotum serves as a sort of air-conditioning structure. Its temperature remains a few degrees lower than the rest of the body, for the sperm cells, which develop inside here, prefer a slightly cooler environment. To maintain the proper temperature, for example, your scrotum tightens up when you are in cold water and stretches if the water is warm. The scrotum also contracts and brings the testicle close to the abdomen when you are frightened or sexually stimulated.

Testicles—The scrotum houses your two testicles (or testes). You can easily feel them with your hand. Each one is about an inch and a half long and about an inch in diameter. They are somewhat oval in shape. Each testicle weighs about half an ounce.

The left testicle usually hangs a bit lower than the right one. So there's nothing to worry about when you see this in your bathroom mirror.

Incidentally, the testicles used to play an important role in the making of an oath. (See Genesis 24:2, 3, 9; 47:29.) In Latin the word *testis* means "a witness." You can now recognize the origin of the verb *testify*. I guess the ancients thought that touching the sex organ would be about as close as one could get to the real center of life. This would provide a strong support for any promise.

Before you were born, your testicles remained inside your body, and just before you entered the world they moved down into your scrotum—but not permanently. In very young boys the testicles can be retracted. For example when you were being trained to use the toilet, you may have watched between your legs to see what was happening. When your stool dropped, your testicles disappeared up into your body at the same time. Some little boys worry that going to the toilet might involve losing their testicles for good. "Down the drain," so to speak.

The testicles create testosterone and sperm cells. Testosterone—a pretty "heavy" word—is a male hormone. It enters the bloodstream and triggers the changes in your body that move you from childhood through adolescence to manhood. Your voice deepens and plays tricks on you, and your body becomes leaner. You grow hair in the genital area, under the arms, and on the face. (You ask, "May I borrow your razor, Dad?")

Your testicles are three-shift factories. They produce sperm cells continuously. It takes from 60 to 70 days for these cells to mature, and your testicles can "create" up to two billion a month. That's somewhere between 20,000 and 70,000 a minute around the clock!

Sometime during this stage of your life the sebaceous glands become overactive and you develop acne. You may want to get help from your doctor or a dermatologist for this bothersome condition. Most often it will respond to medical treatment.

Along with the physical changes that accompany puberty, you also feel an increasing attraction to girls. You begin to wash your neck and ask for clean socks—all without being told. This can be quite a shock to your mother, but a pleasant one. The same girls you once picked on you now like. You tease them in a different way, and they respond in a different way.

Sperm—Back to the production of sperm cells, or spermatazoa. Each sperm has twenty-two chromosomes, plus an X or Y chromosome. The larger and stronger is the X chromosome. Women's ova have only X chromosomes, and when one of these unites with a sperm having a Y chromosome, a baby boy is conceived. (Otherwise a baby girl results.) More boy babies are conceived—about 160 to every 100 girl babies—but more males are spontaneously aborted and more males die in infancy, so females outnumber males in the population at large.

The sperm look like tiny tadpoles, and most of their length is in the tail. They are so small that it takes about 1,200 of them to cover the period at the end of this sentence. Those carrying the X chromosomes have oval-shaped heads and short tails, whereas those carrying the Y chromosomes have round heads and long tails.

Each sperm cell contains thousands of molecules of a chemical called DNA: deoxyribonucleic acid. (You won't use this term very often in your daily conversation!) Each DNA molecule stores a set of chemical directions so complicated and so vast that it is, in a comparative sense, a living computer. These directions form the "blueprint" for the production of a new person. Every cell in your body contains DNA. So you are, in this same sense, a stunning collection of living microscopic "computers."

Semen—Semen is a thick, sticky, whitish fluid made up of liquid and sperm cells. You see, the sperm cells do not have much power to move until they mix with fluids from the prostate gland. Their movement is aided by the contractions of the channels through which they pass and by the wavelike pushing of the cilia (hairlike organs very much like eyelashes) in these tubes.

On their trip to the outer world the sperm first enter the epididymis. Here they mature and then enter a tube called the vas deferens. There are two of these tubes, which open below the bladder and run from the testicles to the seminal vesicles. (In a vasectomy—an operation a man can choose to have to prevent siring any more children—a physician cuts these tubes and ties them off so that no sperm can enter the fluid ejaculated during intercourse.)

At their inner ends the tubes widen into areas called ampullas, which make contact with the seminal vesicles, or pockets. The sperm are stored here for a time, but the vesicles also seem to make the fluid that gives the sperm something to swim in and activates their tail movements.

These two pockets lie behind the prostate gland. This gland may weigh less than an ounce, but it produces the larger part of the fluid a man expels when he ejaculates. The heavily alkaline fluid it makes helps the sperm survive the acid area of the vagina. Otherwise, this part of the trip would destroy most of the sperm cells.

The urethra is a tube that extends from the bladder to the tip of the penis. It carries urine from the bladder when you urinate and prostatic fluid and sperm from the seminal vesicles when you ejaculate. There is no danger of urination, however, during intercourse. The urethra is like a one-track railroad section that carries trains from two lines. When the light is green for one feeder line, the light for the other is red. And only one train can run on the track at any one time. So it is either urination or ejaculation—always one or the other and never both at the same time. You may think it is stupid to mention this, but some young ladies—and young men—do wonder about this.

Most of the seminal fluid is donated by the seminal vesicles, and about a third by the prostate gland. During the average ejaculation about a teaspoonful of semen squirts from the penis.

As you would guess, the brain and the spinal cord have a computerlike tie-in through the nervous system. They program all the operations that mesh together to bring about an effective erection and ejaculation. The whole structure and process is a marvel of divine bioengineering. Biology, physics, chemistry, psychology—all work together in a living man. It's impossible for people like you and me to believe that anyone but God could have designed and created the human sex organs.

Wet Dreams

By the time you turn 14 or 15 you will probably have begun to have wet dreams, or night (nocturnal) emissions. They occur so irregularly that you can hardly predict when you might have one. (If you don't have wet dreams, don't panic—it doesn't mean you're not a man-in-the-making. Some young men rarely—if ever—experience them. Some seminal "tanks" don't seem to build up much pressure.)

After a nocturnal emission you will wake up, perhaps from a pleasant dream involving a young woman, and find your pajamas sticky and wet. At first you might wonder whether you have urinated in your sleep. Then you will notice the small amount of fluid—it could hardly be urine. Besides, it dries quickly into a kind of flakiness. Some think the odor is pleasant; some don't.

When your mother finds this on your pajamas or on the sheet she shouldn't be shocked or disgusted. Instead she'll interpret this as a pretty reliable sign that her son is growing into manhood. After all, your older sister—if you have one—menstruates each month. A wet dream is the nearest we men come to anything like that. But there's nothing regular about it, and there's nothing to wear as "protection," nor is there any reason to worry about it.

In many ways it's unfortunate that we have a double standard when it comes to menstruation and nocturnal emissions. Girls enter early womanhood by menstruation. It's expected and planned for. But fellows have no similar "entry event." We almost sneak into early manhood. Although the onset of nocturnal emissions is roughly equivalent to menarche, we have no similar term for the event, such as "spermarche." Gordan Shipman, after having surveyed four-hundred university students, pointed out that almost one girl in two felt pleased and gratified when her periods began, while only six boys in a hundred had a sense of satisfaction with their evidence of entering manhood.

It is assumed that the pressure of the seminal fluid in the seminal vesicles usually triggers wet dreams. But they are not caused only by an accumulation of secretions. Sexually exciting occasions like indulging in erotic fantasies, reading or looking at pornographic material, or being in the company of a young woman who is particularly "sexy" can also set the stage for a nocturnal emission. Even too tight pajamas can cause them. Once in a while a fellow can bring one on by handling his penis in his sleep. At least it is comforting to know that this activity takes place during the "night shift." It would be awkward, to say the least, if such emissions took place during the day.

However, sperm do not necessarily have to make their exit by way of wet dreams. The body can reabsorb them, but more likely they will find their way out of the body during urination.

The fluid you ejaculate looks quite simple and ordinary, but it contains an amazing variety of substances. Here, for example, are some of them: ammonia, ascorbic acid, calcium, cholesterol, citric acid, lactic acid, magnesium, nitrogen, phosphorus, potassium, sodium, vitamin B_{12}, zinc, copper, and—here's a tongue twister—glycerylphosphorylcholine. (Thanks to Maxwell Roland, M.D., professor of obstetrics and gynecology at French and Polyclinic Medical School, New York City.)

During the previous century many people considered nocturnal emissions to be unhealthy. Many thought that if a young man had them more often than once a month he would injure his health. Medical opinion today strongly disagrees with that idea.

Unfortunately, many of you fellows will not be told about wet dreams. It's too bad that your dads often pass up the opportunity of telling you about these. They often feel too embarrassed to broach the subject, and they assume that you will learn about them in your own way. If you get no advance information the experience of having a wet dream can range from mild surprise to shock, and from an icky feeling to shame.

You might be interested to know that while she sleeps, a woman's vagina "lubricates" itself during some of her dreams. This occurs when she enters the D-periods of sleep (popularly known as REM sleep), which recur four and five times a night. Such experiences are probably the female's counterpart to a male's nocturnal emissions.

Erections

Erections form a part of normal male development. They do not in themselves signify lustful desires or unhealthy thinking, which Christians try to avoid. Spaces in the tissue of the penis can fill with blood and thus become distended or erect. When the blood flows in it makes the penis quite hard or stiff.

Erections can occur during the daytime. Such things as looking at especially stimulating pictures, indulging in a fantasy about a young woman, can trigger an erection. Even friction— like sliding down a rope—can bring one on. Research at Baylor University revealed that normal males have periods of erection during sleep, lasting as long as thirty minutes.

Erections occur fairly frequently. They are part and parcel of maleness. Researchers who have studied fetuses have discovered that even little unborn males can have erections. In the early months of life, male infants often respond to stimulation with erections. (You'll have to admit that this is pretty early, right?)

Exciting thoughts occasionally arise in your mind. A fellow can find himself aroused and even having an erection upon seeing a young woman wearing sexy clothing and engaging in teasing body motions. Such a natural reaction is not in itself sinful. However, should a young man deliberately foster such reactions and try to make them stronger and longer-lasting, then he is moving in the direction of "to lust after," which the Bible condemns. Lust means pushing aside the clean thinking that a Christian conscience expects and letting the senses take over.

Martin Luther is reported to have said that we are not guilty of sin when we let the birds fly over our heads, but we do sin when we permit or encourage them to make nests in our hair!

Worry About Breasts

When some fellows reach puberty their breasts swell a bit and look somewhat like a girl's. In practically every case the condition will disappear within six to eighteen months.

So a young man with this condition does not need to worry about it. It doesn't mean that he is a sissy or that he's a "queer." Some fellows will even try to get out of gym classes because they don't want to undress in front of the other fellows. If you have enlarged breasts and it worries you—especially if your buddies tease you about wearing a bra or taking physical education with the girls—ask your dad to take you to your family doctor for an examination and opinion. Comfort yourself with the knowledge that this can happen to two or three out of five boys around the age of 14 or 15. Enough things in life can complicate the process of growing into maturity, so there's no reason to carry around a secret worry about your breasts.

Hygiene

If you have not been circumcised, when you bathe pull back the foreskin (prepuce) covering the head of your penis and wash the area thoroughly. Also, give special attention to the parts of your body that are special perspiration zones.

If and when you start using aftershave or a men's cologne, don't use too much. Recently in an airport lounge a woman sat down beside me. She was wearing a perfume of such strength that it made me feel overpowered—like a mild gas attack. (And I like some perfumes very much.) Too much of even a good thing can become offensive.

Gentlemanly Christian Conduct

As you read this book you will come across the section on menstruation. You will want to read that section because you need to understand how a girl moves into puberty and what conditions she has to deal with.

Having that knowledge should make you more under-standing and considerate of your mother and sister(s). And when you date young ladies your sensitivity to their needs will make you a more comfortable fellow to be with. When you arrange for a date with your girlfriend there may come times when she will not want to do something you suggest, but she may not wish to tell you why. Often the reason she feels reticent is that her period has started. She will appreciate the fact that you don't keep asking Why?

By now most of you have heard crude names used for the sex organs and their functions. Sometimes people resort to such terms to cover embarrassment, to show off, to give the impression that they are real he-men. Sometimes a person uses such language to give a dirty touch to something funny. You can take it for granted that the names will insult this part of the Lord's creation—which He pronounced "very good" on the sixth day.

Christian young men do not include dirty jokes or stories in their conversation. The Christian gentleman doesn't show or trade suggestive pictures or materials.

Seventh-day Adventist fellows should be the most gentlemanly of all men. A Christian man represents the finest in clean, tender, strong, and protecting manhood. Unfortunately, many young men do not treat young ladies with the respect and consideration they deserve.

One young lady asked in an academy question period: "Why are our guys [SDA] more aggressive and disrespectful than boys who have no religious background?" There are reasons, of course, but no excuses. One reason may be that there are usually more girls than fellows in our churches and academies, so young men feel that with their monopoly on the market they can set their own price for their company. Because Adventist young women are supposed to date and marry only Seventh-day Adventists, Adventist fellows may likely feel little—if any—competition from young men of other faiths.

I would not be fair, however, unless I admitted that some Adventist young ladies don't seem to want to be protected. Because of their aggressive behavior they make it hard for young men to live up to Christian principles. This still doesn't excuse anyone from living up to the ideals that Scripture holds up before us.

I hope you are learning how to relate properly with the women in your home. Christian young men cultivate the virtues of respect, gentleness, tenderness, and fairness. Your mother can serve as a model for those qualities you'd like to see in your future wife. Observing how she relates to your dad can give you an idea as to how a husband and wife should function together in the responsibility and pleasure of marriage. If you have sisters, this will broaden your knowledge of women and make you better able later to relate to the central woman in your life.

Good women look for a man who is loving, who respects them, who is sensitive and tender, yet masculine, who is reasonably intelligent, who can be rough at times, but in a gentle way. And, of course, Adventist women long for a man who truly loves and serves God and who will serve as the "priest" of his future family.

Chapter 6

For the Young Ladies

Anatomy

Breasts—If you are like most maturing girls, when your breasts began to enlarge you felt like a woman. Probably you could hardly wait until you really needed to wear a bra. Teen-age young women sometimes dress in a way to show off their feminine figure, all the while acting as though they are innocent of any intention to do so. Yet, at the same time, they are quite aware of the fellows' reactions.

Your breasts have two functions. Not only do they increase the attractiveness of your figure but they also will serve as milk factories for your babies when you have them. In this latter process, they almost seem to work magic—since they change blood into milk!

One breast, most often the left, is usually a trifle larger than the other. Also, one may hang just a wee bit differently from the other. Breasts contain many sensitive nerve endings, and stimulation by someone you love—husband or baby—can produce pleasant sexual sensations.

Since breasts consist mostly of fat, this is one place where fat is welcome because it actually adds to one's looks. The lover in the Song of Solomon praises his sweetheart's breasts. He compares them to two fawns and to clusters of dates (chaps. 4:5; 7:3, 7, 8, R.S.V.).

The society in which you live frequently acts as though the size of a woman's breasts indicates her sexuality. Yet breast size has very little to do with a woman's capacity for sexual experience. The main center for sexual arousal and response is

55

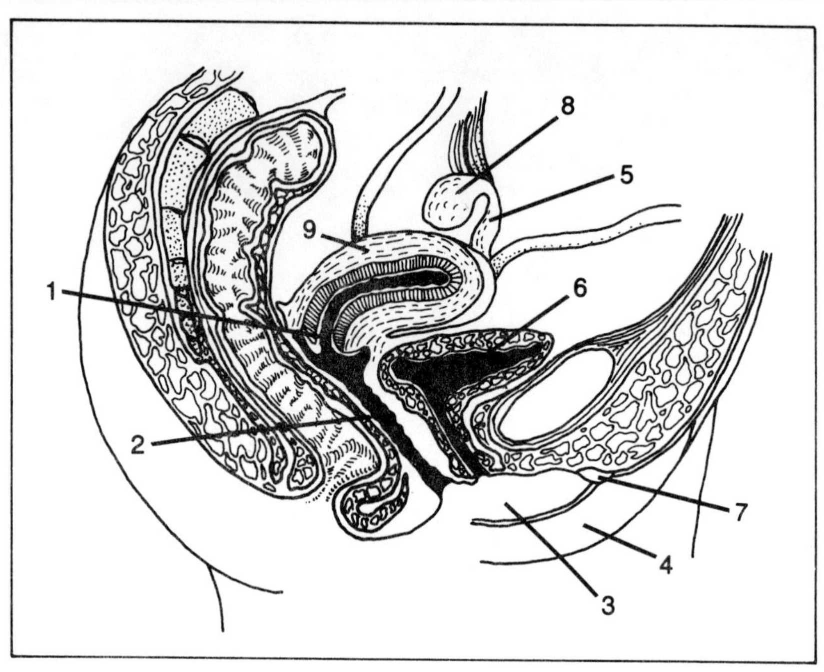

1 cervix

2 vagina

3 inner lip

4 outer lip

5 Fallopian tube

6 bladder

7 clitoris

8 ovary

9 uterus

The female reproductive organs

the brain, not the breasts or genitals.

Contests like the Miss America Pageant have made certain measurements into code numbers for describing a well-shaped young woman. But the modern emphasis on sizable breasts as the mark of sexiness has brought heartache to many women. Some small-breasted women sparkle with magnetic femininity, whereas some large-breasted women quite lack this kind of attraction. Womanliness—femininity—does not depend on physical measurements.

When a man falls in love with you he won't fall in love with just your breasts, but with the whole woman. (I recognize that once in a while a man makes the breasts his particular ideal.) Remember, healthy Christian womanhood lies not in the physically visible organs of the body, but in the physically invisible character and the personality.

Mons—Now let's consider your main sex organs. Where the young man has his scrotum and penis, you have the mons pubis, or mons veneris ("hill of Venus," the goddess of love)—a sort of fleshy mound covered with hair. Your pubic hair indicates sexual maturity. It also acts as a cushion and temperature regulator.

Lips—As you look inward between your thighs (a mirror will make this much easier), you can see the large lips (labia majora) and the small lips (labia minora) running front to back. The large lips consist of folds of skin that are covered generously with pubic hair. The small lips lie between the two larger lips and have no hair.

Inside these lips, on either side of the vagina, are glands that open into this area between the lips. These glands secrete mucus. When a husband and wife make love, this mucus acts as a lubricant to make intercourse more comfortable.

Clitoris—The clitoris protrudes at the point where the small lips meet at the front. In its resting state it may vary from the size of a pea to much larger and still be normal. During intercourse it can erect and become larger. The great number of nerves within the clitoris makes it one of the most sensitive areas of the body, even more sensitive, size for size, than the penis. Before and during intercourse the clitoris acts as the principal trigger to bring on orgasm. Oddly enough, when the clitoris reaches the high point of tension, it tends to pull in. However, the pressure of the penis on the covering of the clitoris and on the area around it continues the pleasant stimulation.

This organ, incidentally, has no other purpose except to make the most intimate act of love a welcome experience, ranging from pleasant to ecstatic. The creation of this little organ gives us an idea of how much happiness and pleasure God intended a woman to have from the sexual act. (In a few cultures, custom unfortunately decrees the removal of the clitoris as a way of decreasing a woman's sexuality.)

Vagina and Hymen—Behind the clitoris, inside the smaller lips and just under the opening to the bladder, lies the opening of the vagina. The hymen, a thin membrane, spans the opening, though it has a passage that allows the menstrual flow to drain off during each period. Presently we know of no particular function for the hymen.

In early Old Testament times if a husband found this membrane ruptured on his wedding night, he assumed that his bride had committed fornication before her marriage. Such an offense drew the death penalty.

The hymen should not provide such an arbitrary test, however, because physical activities, masturbation, the use of tampons, or a medical examination can rupture it. Furthermore, a few girls arrive in the world without one. Some young ladies have such an elastic ring here that they can have intercourse without any noticeable damage to the hymen.

As has been indicated, the hymen acts as a partial door to the vagina. This canal is about three to four inches long. The walls have folds in them that normally touch each other. The whole organ is capable of much enlargement—otherwise a baby could not pass through it at birth.

In intercourse the average penis reaches a length of six inches. (So that you can imagine future intercourse, here is a comparison given by a woman gynecologist. She estimates that it would take about three of the largest tampons to equal the thickness of an erect penis.) If the vagina is three to four inches long, what about the extra three or four inches? Well, you can add about two inches for the lips and outer area. This makes the length of the penis and the length of the vagina about equal. Not only is the vagina very elastic but also the stimulation of intercourse causes it to elongate. Therefore a couple do not need to worry about their genitals not fitting together properly.

The entrance area to the vagina, because of its special concentration of nerves, provides most of the exciting and arousing responses in intercourse. The inner area merely provides the pleasure that comes from a sense of thrusting and fullness.

Cervix—Less than an inch in length and "round like a small doughnut with a tiny hole in the center," the cervix reaches into the vagina. In normal circumstances, a very soft "cork" of mucus keeps it closed—a barrier to possible carriers of infection. It does not discourage the entry of sperm, however. In fact, it helps the sperm onward, for it's easier to swim if you have something to swim in. This slippery condition markedly improves whenever the body expects an egg to be implanted.

Uterus—The uterus, about the shape of a pear, is about three inches long, two inches wide, and an inch thick. Suspended from ligaments, it makes a right angle with the upper end of the vagina. Although the uterus seems very small, it can become hundreds of times larger during pregnancy.

As almost any mother knows, the muscular nature of the uterus comes into full play when a baby makes its entrance into the world. Contractions of three different sets of muscles in the walls of the uterus provide all the labor of moving the infant through the vaginal canal. And these muscles work together in a beautiful rhythm.

Ovaries—The ovaries are connected to the uterus—one on each side. Almond-shaped, they range from half an inch to an inch in length. At birth a baby girl has many thousands of immature eggs already stored in her ovaries. When she matures, one of the ovaries will discharge an egg every twenty-eight to thirty days. Although the eggs (ova) are much larger than the sperm cells, they have no power of their own to move.

In passing, it might interest you to learn that doctors occasionally find teen-age patients (and even adults) who believe that ovaries alternately ovulate and that girl babies come from one side and boy babies from the other. However, such is not the case.

Fallopian Tubes—The Fallopian tubes, narrow fleshy pipes that come off the upper end of the uterus, are several inches long. From them fingerlike projections extend toward the ovaries—almost as if they are trying to reach out for the eggs the ovaries release.

When an ovary discharges an egg, a suctionlike operation draws the egg into the tube nearest that ovary. Once inside the Fallopian tube, the egg is aided in moving toward the uterus by the muscular contractions of the walls of the Fallopian tube and by the wavelike motions of cilia (hairlike parts) within the tube. If a sperm does not fertilize the released egg, the egg is then discharged during menstruation.

Puberty

Many of you have already entered the period known as puberty. The word comes from the Latin *puber*, which means "grown up." Puberty, then, means that you have entered the important stage of becoming an adult.

During puberty your hips broaden, your legs lengthen, and hair appears in your armpits and around the genital area. Hair in the latter area is kinkier than elsewhere and may be called pubes or pubic hair. Also, your breasts begin to swell and the nipples grow more prominent. (Increased nipple sensitivity may require that you take up a different way of dressing.) In general, during puberty your body shape moves from girlish to womanly. The growth usually occurs before you actually menstruate, most of it a year or so before the first flow.

During puberty most young women want information about body hair, breast growth, and acne (pimples that bother some girls a lot in the middle teens). Most teen-age girls find it reassuring to know that breasts don't necessarily develop equally, that menstrual periods do not always come on schedule, and that late maturing is not a socially inferior condition.

Late bloomers should find encouragement in the fact that Sophia Loren, whose figure is world-known, developed quite late. She writes that her friends had enlarged breasts and were menstruating and discussed sexual intercourse and contraception. She pretended she had reached the same level of development, but her body remained skinny. She had flat breasts and had not begun to menstruate. Quite suddenly, however, she began developing very rapidly. Soon she had developed the figure for which she has become known as an actress. (Other women admired for their physical attraction have told similar stories.)

Menstruation

Most young women begin menstruating some time between their tenth and fourteenth birthdays. Within the past century the age of first menstruation (menarche) has dropped at least a year and a half. In the United States the average for the onset of menses falls between 12½ and 13 years. (If you do not begin menstruating by the time you are 15 to 17 years old, you should ask your physician for a thorough examination.) Somewhere between 13 and 15 years of age a young woman can get pregnant if she engages in intercourse.

Late menarche (beginning of menstruation) is not something to worry about or feel embarrassed about. Whether a young lady is on a local or an express, all women arrive at the same station. And since women normally have more than thirty years of menstrual periods ahead of them, they really have lost nothing if they start a bit later than some of their friends. In some cases undernourishment, poor health, or emotional problems can delay the beginning of menstruation.

Fortunately you live in a country and during an era in which menstrual blood is *not* believed to turn wine sour; to kill crops, grafts, and seeds in gardens; to make fruit drop from trees; to cause bees to die; and to drive dogs mad. (From Pliny, with thanks to Elisabeth Connell, M.D.)

You also live in a time when more and more individuals question certain assumptions of the past—such as that women don't function as well as men in intellectual and athletic fields, that women suffer psychological changes because of the menstrual cycle, that hormonal changes cause fluctuations in a woman's emotions.

In the ovaries each egg resides in a follicle, or sac. When the egg matures and is ready to join with a sperm cell, the follicle ruptures and the ovum leaves. Meanwhile, hormones from the brain activate the ovaries to produce estrogen and progesterone. Those hormones in turn prepare the womb to house a fertilized egg and to provide the elements needed for it to grow into a human baby. The lining of the uterus deepens, more blood accumulates in the tissues—it's like a seedbed prepared for planting.

Fertilization takes place if a sperm cell (about one five-hundredth of an inch long—counting its relatively long tail) unites with an egg (about one two-hundredth of an inch in diameter). Out of this union, in about nine months, comes a baby boy or girl.

In their eagerness to reach the egg, the sperm, which have been traveling nonstop from the moment of ejaculation, usually make contact with the ovum about halfway up the Fallopian tube.

Finally one sperm breaks from the pack and dashes in, leaving the rest outside. And the ovum closes the door. Its twenty-three chromosomes become half of those of the fertilized egg. As one girl of twelve wisely remarked, "We are all the result of a winner."

The egg continues on its journey and within three to five days reaches the uterus. It takes another three to five days to embody itself in the wall of the uterus. If a fertilized egg takes up residence in the uterus, then the hormones that prepared the uterus shut down the egg-producing operation in the ovaries. The little beginner receives full priority.

Unfertilized eggs die after a day away from the ovary. Then estrogen and progesterone production drops, and the extra blood and the lining of the uterus are drained away, because they are not needed. (The body treats each potential baby as a special guest, so it keeps no materials as leftovers. Each child begins life with a "nursery" freshly prepared for him or her.) This menstrual fluid consists of blood, cell lining, and a chemical to prevent clotting.

Menstruation is not a dirty process. (You can underline that last sentence.) When you menstruate, you are merely disposing of baby-building materials that you no longer need in this particular cycle. (In the course of a normal lifetime a woman's ovaries will ripen four hundred to five hundred eggs. She has a generous reserve supply—vastly more than she could ever need.)

Many of you young ladies reading this have already begun to menstruate. You have chosen between a napkin and a tampon to absorb the flow during your period. (Napkins collect the flow on the outside of the vagina. Tampons collect it on the inside.) Most young women find napkins easier to use to begin with. First insertion of a tampon sometimes requires the assistance of your mother or sister, or an office or school nurse. One obstetrician tells me that he and his colleagues do not recommend using tampons until at least one year after the onset of menses.

If you prefer using tampons you will probably want to start with a junior size and choose those with lubricated tips. Since they are tapered and no larger than your middle finger, you can quickly feel comfortable using them.

The 1980 *Buying Guide Issue* of *Consumer Reports* evaluates menstrual tampons and pads. About 4,500 women participated and rated many brands. The general finding: "More women seemed more satisfied with tampons than with conventional pads." More than two hundred of the women wrote that their doctors had warned them not to use deodorant tampons or pads. This is "because of the possibility of an irritating or allergic reaction."

If you use tampons you will probably gain a good idea of the structure of part of your sexual organs. Tampons also make it easier for you to imagine what intercourse will be like. In fact, the use of tampons stretches the hymen and thus makes the first intercourse with your husband more free from discomfort.

In late 1980 the news media called attention to a disease known as toxic-shock syndrome. The Center for Disease Control in Atlanta stated that several hundred women had suffered from this staph-type disease and that about 10 percent had died. A year later estimates of death rose to 80 individuals. Tampon manufacturers were to meet on January 6, 1982, to adopt standards for the industry.

A spokesman for the American College of Obstetricians and Gynecologists advised women to avoid using superabsorbent tampons. A fiber in these seems to have been the villain. In addition, the same group of doctors recommended that women "change tampons at least every six to eight hours and that they use sanitary napkins or minipads during the night."

One television news bulletin (December, 1980) referred to toxic-shock syndrome as an "extremely rare ailment." By the time you read this your physician will know much more about this disease and can advise you about the use of tampons.

Some women suffer from tension before their menstrual period begins. Some contract cramps, backache, and pelvic discomfort. They tend to feel jumpy and irritable and to get the blues. Perhaps the pressure of held-back salt and water causes the feelings. If you suffer from cramps, talk to your physician. He can prescribe anticramp medications.

The normal menstrual period runs from three to five days and results in the loss of one to three ounces of blood. One physician estimates that the average period requires the use of ten to fifteen pads or tampons.

Incidentally, the interval between periods can vary from woman to woman. In the same family one girl may menstruate every 24 days, while her sister takes the full 28 days or more. A normal interval, in the broad sense, ranges from 21 to 35 days. Other things being equal, regularity is more important than the particular length of time between periods.

Emotions, especially stress, can affect the regularity of the menstrual cycle. My wife, two girls, and I spent more than three years in a Japanese internment camp. Many of the women incarcerated there stopped menstruating because of the stress, the poor diet, and the depressing living conditions.

Good health habits will help you maintain normal menstrual periods. Posture, muscle tone, kinds of food eaten, eating habits, amount of sleep—all can play a part in providing you with comfortable menstrual periods.

By all means see your doctor if your periods show too much irregularity, or if you feel that the flow is too heavy or too little, or if you have pains or unusual discharges between periods, or if you experience marked changes in your cycle.

Since you will menstruate many times before your marriage, you will become familiar with your body clock. By careful calculations you will be able to set a wedding date so that you will not have a menstrual period on your honeymoon. You may want to begin keeping your own menstrual calendar.

The Old Testament lists intercourse during the wife's menstrual period among the abominations that defiled the land of Canaan before the Israelites arrived. The abominable practices included bestiality, incest, and homosexuality. (See Lev. 18:19-24.) Anyone who engaged in intercourse during a woman's menstrual period was cut off from the people. (I don't know how the authorities could have known who did so.)

Ezekiel classifies intercourse during menstruation with idolatry, adultery, oppression, and spoilation by violence and usury (Eze. 18:6-8). A man who lives in a lawful and right way will abstain, he writes.

Many Christians feel that they should continue to abide by these restrictions. Dr. William Fitch, a Presbyterian minister and writer on the subject of sex and marriage, says: "There is a normal monthly period when a woman because of menstrual flow can not countenance sexual relations." He estimates that menstruation at the outset of a honeymoon happens about seventeen times out of a hundred and advises against beginning sexual relations at such a time. He feels that the couple then can take time to adjust by having a more relaxing relationship. (*Christian Perspective on Sex and Marriage*, pp. 77, 78.)

I discuss this topic at more length in *God Invented Sex*. You and your husband will come to your own decision in this matter. I think most conservative Christians abstain from intercourse during such periods. Others may abstain because they assume it is not the nice thing to do or because they feel that a sensitive husband would not expect his wife to allow such intimate lovemaking during menstruation.

Although a bride tries to set her wedding date so that she will not have a menstrual period at that time, sometimes a change in her rhythm throws off the arithmetic. For the couple this means an unwelcome delay of intercourse. She may, under such circumstances, enjoy relieving her husband's sexual tensions by caressing his penis and bringing him to ejaculation. He in turn will doubtless find it pleasurable to stimulate by hand her clitoral area. (You should not confuse this practice with masturbation.)

Sometimes circumstances dictate that the wedding has to fall on a certain date. If it appears likely that the bride's period will occur at that time, a young woman, with the help of her physician and the use of oral contraceptives, can delay the onset of her period until after the honeymoon.

When the time of your wedding nears, you may feel a bit nervous about how you will do on the first night. As one bride-to-be put it, "I've often wondered how to approach my soon-coming wedding night. We want to make God first in our lives. What should we do when we get to our destination? Have family worship? and then the 'normal' follows? As I think about it, it seems that I'll be awkward."

Having family worship is the sound and happy way to begin life together. Both of you will be tired, but you, the bride, much more. The weight of planning the wedding has fallen on you and your family. Sometimes a chase after the reception adds to the fatigue of the day. Yet, if you both still want to engage in sex the first night, there is certainly no reason why you shouldn't. However, if you decide that you are too tired to get the most out of the first experience in sex, your husband may gallantly offer to wait until you have rested a bit and have become more used to such intimate circumstances. And sex in the morning would be a delightful way to begin the first full day of marriage!

What the young lady calls "awkward" is not a fair way of describing inexperience—especially inexperience that is a credit to her and to him. Learning together—even fumbling a bit—at the start can be enjoyable. It doesn't take long to learn the basics of intercourse, and you have all the long years ahead (God willing) to acquire additional skills and to deepen your sexual involvement and communication.

Hygiene

Lorna and Philip Sarrel, of Yale, point out that the increase in circulating estrogen during puberty causes most young women to have a vaginal discharge. Naturally, such a condition can arouse much anxiety and embarrassment. The Sarrels recommend that the subject should be included as part of sex education and as part of a girl's medical history. (See *Sexual Unfolding, Sexual Development and Sex Therapies in Late Adolescence*, pp. 23, 24.)

Obviously, you want to guard against body odor. Bacteria work on perspiration and body secretions, especially in those parts that are usually warm and moist. The covering of the clitoris can accumulate secretions that if not removed can cause odor or make the foreskin adhere. (If they are not circumcised, men have to guard against a similar condition.) Clothing that hugs the genital areas too closely can increase the possibility of the development of an unpleasant odor or can encourage the growth of germs and fungi.

Advertising makes the douche seem almost a must in the life of the fastidious woman. However, medical authorities feel that many women should not find it necessary to douche. A healthy vagina lubricates itself and cleans itself. Seminal fluid deposited in the vagina during intercourse does not need to be removed because it is normally germ-free. Most of the semen will flow spontaneously out of the vagina. In addition, the vagina is self-cleansing.

Ladylike Christian Conduct

Nearly all of you will fit into the category of attractive. Some of you can be called pretty, whereas only a very few, beautiful. Similarly only a very few men are handsome. A fair number are good-looking. Obviously, then, most people do not marry just for looks. Other things count heavily: character, personality, friendliness, warmth, caring, intelligence, and spiritual maturity.

A woman's great attractiveness and seductiveness (in the right sense) lies in the appearance of her femininity. (Don't confuse this with sexiness, which exaggerates the physical features of sex and capitalizes on certain subtle overtones of suggestiveness and attention-getting behavior.) In friendship and courting days, therefore, one should not place the main emphasis on what we commonly term sex appeal. Character and personality are the main factors of value in the long run. Sexual (physical and emotional) attraction, of course, can be "icing on the cake"—but it is not the cake itself.

Clothing becomes a consideration in this connection. Although young men have to bear the responsibility for their impure thoughts, young women share a measure of guilt if they dress and behave provocatively. Clothing that exposes too much or unduly emphasizes the breasts, buttocks, or the genital area—with conduct to match—makes it easier for a fellow to assume that the young lady is giving him subtle signals of her availability.

Genuine love far surpasses mere sexual attraction. Dr. Joyce Brothers points out some fringe benefits of love: increased physical attractiveness, more erect carriage, shinier eyes, faster-beating heart, improved health, and more energy. Real love has a healthy effect on the whole body and personality. I often tell women with serious marriage problems that when we have put the marriage on a happy level they will look five years younger. And when things are better, even their husbands walk with a springier step, smile easier, and seem to "purr" oftener!

On the purely practical side, I'd like to urge you to postpone marriage until you have reached a level of education that will allow you to work at a job that can bring a reasonable amount of financial return. Remember, however, that there is no higher calling than that of devoted wife and mother.

Chapter 7

Sleeping Double in a Double Bed

After the wedding service most couples go on a honeymoon—in the mountains, on the beach, or traveling to special places. Some, because of work obligations, have to honeymoon quite close to home. A few couples even celebrate their honeymoon at home.

Most couples have intercourse their first night together. You can be sure that the husband has looked forward to this first sex for months and has now reached a high level of eagerness and anticipation. Most brides also eagerly anticipate sexual intimacy, but usually in a less physically intense way.

The First Night

On the first night some brides feel a bit shy about undressing in front of their husband, so they change into their night clothes in the bathroom. Most likely this is the first time they have worn a filmy nightgown or a satiny one that invites touch, with the intention to please and excite. Perfume may add to the mood. (Note Song of Solomon 5:4, 5.) It is also the first occasion (I am assuming virginity here) they have gone to bed with a man. However, with a sort of pleasant nervousness and self-consciousness, most newlyweds quickly adjust to this new situation. The bride wants to be sure that when later he sees her naked for the first time he will be delighted with what he sees.

Some brides do not feel emotionally ready for intercourse on the first night. They are suffering from the drained feeling that comes from the fairly long and heavy pressure of the wedding preparations. Even though a wedding is a wonderful event and a memory to savor the rest of her married life, it does demand a large investment of emotional and physical energy. Naturally, the tension multiplies many times over if anything goes wrong at the wedding: unexpected delays, last-minute changes, embarrassing conduct of any wedding guests, too much and too noisy attentions during the "getaway."

Now that they are alone together, the husband's tact and self-control will count for a lot in the attitude his wife develops toward the sexual part of their marriage. Upon going to bed, the husband and wife may talk awhile on personal matters that the day's tight schedule did not allow them to share. Gradually they ease into lovemaking, which usually leads up to intercourse. We call this special lovemaking foreplay—playing before.

Foreplay

They kiss, nuzzle, tease, caress different parts of the body, sometimes even bite lightly. The husband gently strokes his wife's clitoris or, if it is a bit tender, the area around it. One woman specialist in sexuality puts it more strongly by saying that it is imperative that the head of the clitoris not be touched directly. The clitoris, in a sense, is the starter button for orgasm. She, in turn, will stroke his penis in any intimate way that appeals to him and to her. (Occasionally a woman takes a little time to get used to fondling her husband's penis. If she has had no sex education or the wrong kind, she may believe that women don't touch a man *there*—that it is an unclean activity or the same thing as masturbation.)

Sometimes a Christian wife worries about taking too active a part in foreplay. Perhaps she hesitates for fear of arousing her husband's animal passions. But if she has a balanced and wholesome understanding of sex, she soon learns to enjoy this part of lovemaking. And as she loses herself in love-play, she finds her own ardor rising in response to the obvious signs of his tension and eagerness.

Foreplay is very much like warming up an engine or priming a pump. (You girls will forgive me for using such a "mechanical" illustration.) It provides the main preparation for a woman's orgasm. This has a lot to do with the speed of response on a woman's part. In fact, orgasm often occurs during foreplay.

Husbands and wives lay the foundation for sexual expression by the way they treat each other in the morning and the afternoon and the evening of each day. Loving behavior should always proceed intercourse. Many husbands seem unaware of this. They expect their wives at night to approach lovemaking eagerly even if they have received no conditioning for it.

Women are not sexually aroused as quickly as are men. And the length of time it takes for a woman to reach orgasm varies. Some couples like to make the foreplay period long: thirty or forty minutes. Most can reach the final point in less time. The amount of time spent is not an important factor. It is important, however, to do whatever best suits the particular sexual rhythm of the couple. Intercourse is not a form of athletics. Couples should not embark on it with a checklist in one hand and a stopwatch in the other.

Foreplay typically lasts from a few minutes to twenty minutes or more. A short time period suffices when both feel in a keyed-up mood and eagerly desire a quick result. Most lovemaking, however, requires a longer period of time.

The Act of Intercourse

During foreplay the husband's penis quickly erects, and he has reached the point of tension necessary for penetration. As has been mentioned and odd as it may seem, smaller penises proportionately increase in size more than larger penises. Thus men are much more alike in penile size at the finish line than they are at the start of the race. This should comfort any husband who worries about the size of his penis.

The wife ordinarily takes longer to reach a corresponding point of tension. When she feels ready to go on to the next part, she tells him or signals him with her hand. She lies on her back and spreads her legs apart, with her knees up. She may rest her hips on a pillow for greater comfort and pleasure. The man lies above her and inside her legs. She may guide his penis into the vagina with her hand.

The husband supports himself on his elbows—otherwise a heavy man may just about smother his wife. (You have probably wondered about that when you have seen a tall and heavy husband with his small and lightweight wife.) He then thrusts his penis up and down, back and forth, fast or slowly, roughly or gently, shallowly or deeply—depending on their mood at the time. The enclosed feeling of the vagina on his penis titillates the husband. And the sensation of his firm penis moving within her body is delightfully pleasing to the wife. The male and female sensations complement each other.

During the extended period of lovemaking, the bodies of both the man and the woman undergo specific and predictable changes. In building up to orgasm or an equivalent feeling, the wife's pulse rate and blood pressure rise. Parts of the body may be flushed, and she will breathe faster and deeper. The clitoris becomes erect. The muscles tense.

The vagina, sensitive to the feeling of penetration and pressure of the penis, stretches and becomes longer. At the same time, lubrication readies the vagina for the penis. The vagina "sweats," and the glands in the lips produce mucus (I don't care for this word) that's pretty much like the saliva in our mouths. Lubrication usually increases proportionately to the level of excitement. Some wives produce less lubrication than the average, but this doesn't mean they do not love their husbands or their attentions. Extra help is available for these women in the form of a jelly made especially for this purpose. (One brand is known as KY Jelly.) Vaseline, because it is not water-soluble, is a poor choice.

The ring muscle at the viginal opening grips the penis and increases the sensation of friction. The contractions of the vaginal muscles tease the penis into staying erect and firm. (In some women these contractions are quite slight.)

The woman's nipples will (some say, may) erect, and her breasts will become larger. The uterus also takes part in the activity, and as the level of excitement rises, it raises itself out of the pelvis. During orgasm the contracting pattern that it develops resembles that occurring in early stages of labor.

Orgasm

As the husband builds to ejaculation, his body experiences some of the same changes. In addition, his penis becomes larger and harder—very much like firming up a tire. The erection is produced by blood flowing into the cavities of the penis and being blocked from going out by sphincter muscles. The testes rise a little and may enlarge quite a bit. The skin of the scrotum thickens. Cowper's glands add a little secretion. Meanwhile seminal fluid collects in the prostate area and in the urethra. Contractions in the prostate gland, the seminal vesicles, the vas deferens, the renal sphincter, the bladder, and the urethra (quite a lineup!) all work together to drive the seminal fluid through the penis. The fluid is shot out into the vagina at the mouth of the uterus. Called an ejaculation, this is the climax of intercourse for a man.

The sensation of expelling seminal fluid is one of the most exciting feelings that a man can experience. Usually he experiences a few strong surges that then fade off into weaker ones. Following ejaculation, every organ involved relaxes, the blood leaves the penis, and it becomes limp, or flaccid.

Some husbands try very hard to keep the penis in contact with the clitoris during insertion and the ensuing climax. But this is rather difficult to do. Such direct contact is not really necessary, since the clitoris reacts to the stimulation going on all around it and by the pressures against it. As a matter of fact, when a woman's excitement reaches a high level, her clitoris pulls in and flattens itself. It almost seems to turn bashful as the high level of excitement gets nearer.

During her orgasm the wife will not ejaculate any fluid, but she will feel a series of muscular contractions that occur about a second apart. She also enjoys a lot of accompanying sensations that are well-nigh impossible to describe. Orgasm can be out of this world or just a delightful relaxation of tension. One woman has observed that they can vary like the difference between a light sneeze and one that shakes the walls!

The wife's orgasm and the husband's ejaculation do not have to occur at the same time. In fact, there are definite advantages if one partner does precede the other. Each can then give full attention to what is happening to the other. And that's a big part of the pleasure of lovemaking—enjoying the spouse's joy and being excited by the spouse's excitement.

(For the comfort of husbands who come early, they should know that many men reach ejaculation in two minutes or less. Probably seven men out of ten ejaculate in less than ten minutes. These figures can reassure any man who may feel guilty for moving too fast, though premature ejaculation can prove very frustrating to a woman left with unfulfilled sexual desires and tensions.)

Sometimes the wife will reach orgasm during her husband's manual stimulation of the clitoral area. This orgasm is just as real as the one experienced when he is inside her.

Occasionally, orgasm or ejaculation does not occur at all for one of the parties, but the lovemaking can still prove deeply satisfying. Neither the husband nor the wife should feel obliged to produce an orgasm every time. If the husband feels that this is a must, the whole action becomes more like trying to reach a goal in a game. Being totally at ease with each other, tuned in on the mood of the moment, and wanting to give as much pleasure to each other as possible will make any time of lovemaking completely satisfying to both marriage partners.

Some young people develop unrealistic expectations about sex. You need to recognize that you won't always "go into orbit" during intercourse. Highly titillating sex is not like getting an A for every class taken. The emotional response varies from time to time, so a strong B average would probably indicate that you enjoy a very satisfying sex life. Couples need to allow for highs and lows and mediums.

After I had made this qualified statement about the level of pleasure and excitement in intercourse, this note came to me in the period devoted to questions: "My dear Doctor W: Question: Do you think that you may have misspoken last evening? If I recall correctly, you said that a wife or a husband should not expect the bells to ring, to bat 1,000, to see Roman candles, to see stars, to hear whistles, to feel like the Fourth of July—every time. But I do! What am I doing wrong? Your humble, obedient, and waiting student." (The name was signed.)

Both she and her husband, friends of mine, had recently entered a second marriage, which, in each case, was vastly better than the one preceding. This gentle and humorous dissent is largely due to that circumstance, I feel.

However, at another meeting a man sent in this comment: "My wife and I are in our mid-fifties, and we have 'homers' all the time! Can you explain this?"

These reports are delightful, but I still think that my more conservative description fits most marriages.

Some women enjoy intercourse deeply although they do not experience orgasm. In *God Invented Sex*, I reported on a study of more than 2,000 married women who were asked, "Of all aspects of sexual activity, what do you like best?" Only 21 percent said, "Orgasm." About one in five favored the act of intercourse, or the feeling of closeness and oneness, or the foreplay. Many people have discovered that they should not try too hard for an orgasm. Individuals who try too hard often find that orgasm can be very elusive. Orgasms are much more likely to "sneak up" on you if you just let yourself go and revel in the excitement and stimulation of intercourse.

Generally speaking, a wife takes longer than her husband to reach that level of sexual tension which readies one for intercourse. A caring wife, however, sometimes engages in intercourse when she does not feel in the mood for it, just to please the husband. (And vice versa.) This is one way of showing what Paul meant when he wrote that in marriage each partner's body belongs to the other. Notice, however, that I wrote, "sometimes." To regularly have intercourse just to satisfy the spouse turns lovemaking into a service rather than a shared and welcome experience.

As both partners build up to the climax, they should be careful lest they break the rhythm. This is not a time for distractions. Any interruption can slow down the buildup of sexual tensions to the point where—using an auto term—the engine stalls. It's hardly the time to ask where the cat is, or whether the light in the garage is off.

After intercourse the thoughtful and sensitive husband shows his wife any attentions that will help her return to normal as happily and comfortably as she can. Not only does a woman build slowly to climax, but also her sexual tensions release more slowly than do a man's. Some couples like to stay in each other's arms for a while, and some even enjoy falling off to sleep this way. In comparison with foreplay, this aspect might be called the afterplay or afterglow. Many women enjoy the afterplay almost as much as they do the act of intercourse. They wind down more slowly than their husbands and find it delightful to have their loving attention in the process.

Will It Hurt?

Any young bride whose hymen is still intact will feel a little stab of pain when her husband penetrates her for the first time. This is a one-time pain, because of the tearing of the hymen, but in the excitement and pleasure of the moment many wives hardly notice it. If before marriage you feel that your hymen may cause difficulty and more-than-usual pain during the first intercourse, you can ask your doctor to refer you to a gynecologist, who can provide you with a hymen stretcher.

If you are a young woman, don't worry about pain or discomfort as you look ahead to coitus and wonder whether your husband's penis will be too large. The human sex organs that do the actual connecting are like gloves or socks made to fit all sizes. Since the vagina can accommodate itself to a baby's head, it can easily and comfortably welcome a man's erect penis.

If a woman has pain during intercourse, she might have a physical disorder. (Every young woman should undergo a complete physical before her wedding day. It wouldn't hurt men to have the same.) Most commonly, though, and unconscious fear brings on spasms in the muscles around the entrance to the vagina, which triggers the pain. This can happen even when she really wants to enjoy sex. For help in overcoming such a problem, she will need to consult a marriage counselor or sex therapist. Fortunately, relatively few young wives ever encounter such trouble.

Technique

Perhaps I should include a few words about sexual techniques. Techniques certainly have their place, but any lovemaking that is guided by sensitivity, caring, wholesome passion, and reasonable intelligence can hardly fail to please. Couples have years in which to learn each other's preferences and to develop richly satisfying ways of making love. (When I write, "years," I'm not forgetting that our Lord's coming may be nearer than we think.)

As you approach your wedding day, you may want to buy one of the popular books on Christian marriage that relate detailed information about these matters. Three of the currently available are: *The Compleat Marriage* by Nancy Van Pelt (SDA), *The Act of Marriage* by Tim and Beverly La Haye, and *Intended for Pleasure* by Ed and Gaye Wheat.

The introduction in the book jacket of *Intended for Pleasure* states that "God himself [sic] invented sex." (I am using this *sic* to indicate no capital for *himself*, OK?) Which brings me to another suggestion. If you are in the later academy or high school years and want to expand your "theology of sex," you might like to read my first book, *God Invented Sex*, which appeared in 1974, and is still in print. Many teen-agers have already read it.

Couples can use different positions for intercourse, three are the most popular. The first I have already described—the husband lies above his wife.

In another popular position the wife takes the astride position. She lies above her husband and does practically all the moving. In this way she can make the contact with the penis that best stimulates her. Most husbands I have dealt with get an extra gleam in their eyes when this is suggested in marriage counseling—sometimes to the surprise of their wives. Many husbands get an extra charge out of having the wife take a more active role. Besides, the position gives the man a better opportunity to fondle her breasts.

In the third position, the husband enters the vagina from behind his wife. The bodies in this configuration somewhat resemble a spoon within a spoon. Couples often choose the rear entry position during the later stages of pregnancy. There are other positions, of course, but this is enough by way of introduction.

The previous discussion will suffice to help you imagine the sexual pleasures that lie ahead and to understand now the ultimate functions of your sexual organs. Surely they are a marvel of "bioengineering," both in themselves and in the way they complement each other. I, for one, simply cannot grasp how evolution could in any way even remotely stumble on the design and function of these amazing organs. And this without saying anything about the marvelous emotional sharing that sex makes possible. The God of Creation surely implied a great deal when He ended the first wedding service with the words "And they shall be one flesh."

Should a husband and wife want to make love but do not plan for a child, they can use a number of methods to prevent the sperm from reaching the ovum. As you move closer to marriage you can decide what method you wish to use.

If the husband does not prevent conception by wearing a condom, then the wife can keep a small towel or handkerchief under her pillow to absorb the small amount of seminal fluid that drains out after intercourse. If the wife wishes to become pregnant she sometimes maintains a position that will help her retain the semen for a longer time so the chance of fertilization can become much greater.

How often do couples engage in intercourse? It all depends on the desires of the couple, the sex drives of both, the state of health and energy, the bedroom conditions, et cetera. Most young people (and many older) enjoy intercourse two or three times a week. Sometimes a couple celebrating a special occasion will have sex that frequently within a day—a wedding anniversary, the husband's return after a long absence, or the beginning of a vacation in a romantic spot.

You may have heard through the years that a woman surrenders herself to a man in intercourse. But the word *surrender* does not appropriately express what happens in loving intercourse. Actually, both husband and wife give themselves wholly to each other. Both are, by invitation and desire, totally in control of the other. God intended sexual intercourse to provide the most intimate kind of knowing. It is not surrender, but a sharing together in the most personal kind of intimacy.

Chapter 8

"Male and Female Created He Them"

When Jesus appeared on earth as a man, He assumed the nature and personality of a strong masculine person. He engaged in a trade requiring muscle. With His disciples He hiked many miles, sometimes sleeping out overnight in the open air. We cannot but admire His supreme courage and selflessness in the final days of His life. Indeed, the cross is the ultimate symbol of true manhood.

Several of the men He chose to accompany Him belonged to the fraternity of fishermen—men whose work, of necessity, called for ruggedness. In addition, He selected Levi-Matthew, once a hard-bitten tax collector, and Simon the Zealot, formerly a fiery, uncompromising Roman-hater. Surely, Jesus' company of disciples contained no man whose sexual orientation was in any degree in doubt.

Our commitment to the Lord includes abstinence from smoking and drinking. It means leaving out of the life questionable dancing and music and any entertainment unsuitable for Christians. Christian Seventh-day Adventists also generally avoid the world's too intense interest in sports.

Because of these conditions, fellows are sometimes tempted to think that our religion makes them less masculine, less regular guys. But activities such as those just mentioned never produce or prove masculinity (in spite of the beer and cigarette ads you see)!

Consider the following brief quotations:

The influence of most athletic sports "does not tend toward refinement, generosity, or real manliness" (*Education*, p. 210).

"The only way in which any can be secure against the power of intemperance is to abstain wholly from wine, beer, and strong drinks. We must teach our children that in order to be manly they must let these things alone. God has shown us what constitutes true manliness."—*Child Guidance*, p. 401.

"Let everyone who professes Christ seek to overcome all unmanliness, all weakness and folly."—*Testimonies*, vol. 5, p. 597.

The same holds true for womanliness. Notice:

"Manliness, womanliness—sanctified, purified, refined, ennobled—we have the promise of receiving."—*Selected Messages*, book 1, p. 88.

"Girls should be taught that the true charm of womanliness is not alone in beauty of form or feature, nor in the possession of accomplishments; but in a meek and quiet spirit, in patience, generosity, kindness, and a willingness to do and suffer for others. They should be taught to work, to study to some purpose, to live for some object, to trust in God and fear Him, and to respect their parents. Then as they advance in years, they will grow more pure-minded, self-reliant, and beloved. It will be impossible to degrade such a woman. She will escape the temptations and trials that have been the ruin of so many."—*Child Guidance*, p. 140.

And here's the clincher:

"All that makes men manly or women womanly is reflected from the character of Christ."—*Counsels to Parents and Teachers*, p. 541.

Sex Appeal

True sex appeal springs from Christian manliness and womanliness. Sex is what you are—in the sense that your own sexuality is a component of every aspect of your body and your personality. You can't separate your sexness from the rest of you. It is not confined to your sex organs, nor does it disappear with age (even though, in men, their ability to engage in intercourse may wane in late age).

Furthermore, sex appeal is not based primarily on looks. Certainly this comes as a cheering fact, since most of us do not have dream bodies. All the qualities that make up a fine personality are factors in attraction. (Incidentally, no one *has* a personality. Each individual *is* a personality.) The kind of person you are spiritually, emotionally, and socially plays a big part in someone's choosing you as a sweetheart and potential mate.

Sex Education

It is almost as easy to get a marriage license as it is to get a dog license. No preparation or training period—as in driver education, for example—is required. Marriage is easy to enter and difficult—even painful— to leave.

Sex education can play a large part in helping you see yourself as a sexual person. It can point out that copulation is not of itself lovemaking. It should teach that intercourse at its best is love finding physical expression at the most intimate level.

Sex education can help you understand the risks and advantages, the pleasures and sorrows, possible in a sexual relationshp. It can also help you understand better those persons who don't travel the normal road of sexual fulfillment.

Some people assume that sex education means finding out all about sex and how people "do it." Actually, learning the main points of anatomy and the mechanics of intercourse does not take long. As to the purely physical aspect of sex, any intelligent fellow or girl can get the know-how in a very short time. But it can take years of living together and loving to acquire the maturity of spirit and emotion that will give the process of lovemaking its God-intended feeling and meaning.

You can understand the basics of riding a bicycle in just a minute or two, but it usually takes hours of practice before the theory becomes real so that you can ride with skill. You can learn about driving a car from a very brief lecture with diagrams and illustrations, but again you must spend months acquiring the habit patterns that will make you a safe driver. Similarly, the capacity to love your future husband or wife as Christ loves the church is not acquired except by long, and sometimes painful, experience.

The important elements of real love—devotion, caring, communication, acceptance, genuine liking, commitment— take a lifetime of cultivation and practice. A happy marriage represents a lifetime of cultivation and practice. A happy marriage represents a lifelong blending of two different persons in all aspects of their natures. This was symbolized in the Edenic marriage service by God's words "And you shall be one flesh."

The Sex Drive

Neither a young man nor a young woman is at the mercy of the sex drive. You need not be forced into wrong sexual behavior to relieve tension. Channeling your energies into other activities is one way to control pressure at peak periods.

Sex is like a horse, a spirited horse. You don't want him to throw you, but you don't want to lock him in the barn or drug him. He's there to be ridden, controlled, and enjoyed. Abusing him, misusing him, losing control, does away with the fun of having him.

When fellows enter puberty, they experience a strong sex drive and a great interest in sexual activity. Teen-age girls normally move much more slowly in this area. If we make a comparison, young men's sexual interests go up at a sharp angle and at high speed, whereas young ladies' sex drives advance on a long, slow curve. At least this has been the case up to the present time, but changing attitudes on the part of women may alter this comparison.

The Christian depends on his close relation to the Lord, his instant access in prayer, and his profound desire to do nothing that would displease his Lord. Every Christian understands the meaning of Joseph's rebuke to Potiphar's wife when she tried to seduce him: "How . . . can I do this great wickedness, and sin against God?"

Isn't Sex Dirty?

Unfortunately, many people still think of sex as dirty. Probably one reason they do so is the association people make as a result of their early toilet training.

Remember when you were little? You were playing outside on a warm spring day. Soon you would have your turn at being the leader in the game, but you needed to urinate. Since you didn't want to lose your place in the game, you took care of your natural need right there. It didn't bother you, and didn't bother your friends. (They would most likely be doing the same thing soon themselves!) But your mother happened to look out the window just at the right moment. She stormed out of the house and said, "Oh, no, not again! Why didn't you call Mommy and tell her you needed to go to the bathroom?" (Or whatever expression she used for this function.) Then she marched you inside to the bathroom and told you firmly that next time you must let her know. Somehow you got the impression that you had done something dirty—it surely must be because you always ended up in this particular room for cleaning.

Somehow, during this period of toilet training, parents often forget to remind their children that their sex organs are clean. The penis discharges urine, which is just a sterile waste product of the body machinery. The same, of course, is true of the girl's urethra. The vagina, a close neighbor, is also clean—in fact, probably cleaner than most people's mouths!

Furthermore, the divine love, wisdom, and power revealed in the creation of the eye, the heart, the stomach, and the brain are equally evident in the creation of the sex organs. They are just as marvelous examples of body engineering as any other organ.

The sex organs deserve the same respect we have for other parts of the body. We do not keep the sex organs covered because they are dirty, but because we consider them and their functions to be private. Jesus Himself had the body of a human male, thus honoring the body that He Himself had made and called "very good."

Whenever we sexually misbehave, it is the mind that sins and not the sexual organs. No part of the body except the mind is accountable for sin. Therefore, we should not accuse certain organs of sin when the brain urges them to do something wrong. We sin as thinking, volitional human beings.

Another reason some individuals feel that sex is bad comes as a result of having gotten caught in sex play with another child. Probably many of you tried to play doctor with a neighbor boy or girl. When your parents discovered what you were playing, they got pretty disgusted and angry. From the way they jumped on you, you got the impression that this part of your body was not nice to look at or play with. They were right, of course, in discouraging sex play, but sometimes unwise in the way they went about it. (Perhaps your parents handled this very well.) So some youngsters pick up the feeling that their parents forbade this activity because their sex organs are dirty and their childish curiosity is bad.

Since society generally regards as dirty those magazines and books that cater to prurient interests by capitalizing on sex, young people may assume that the genitals and the act of sexual intercourse are somehow inherently dirty. They fail to realize that it is the distortion and exploitation of sex that make these publications dirty—or lewd.

Changing Feelings Toward Each Other

You young men during your early preteen years experienced different feelings about girls than you do now. Back then you thought they were too clean, too goody-goody. They were tattletales and nuisances.

You young ladies considered boys to be noisy, dirty, rough, crude. They even carried snakes and frogs in their pockets and wrestled in the dirt.

Now that the male hormone has made its impact on you fellows and the female hormone has done its work in you young women, you regard each other more kindly—in fact, you sense a definite desire to enjoy each other's company.

The boy who used to pull your hair and throw snowballs at you is now the young man who walks you to school. Whereas he once gave you a yukky feeling, you now get a thrill in his company.

Have you noticed how the atmosphere changes when a good-looking fellow joins two young ladies who are chatting together? Or when two fellows are just "standing around" and a pretty girl moves into their twosome? That's the result of the hormones too. As some of you might put it, the vibes are different.

Infatuation

What teens usually term *love* is often *infatuation*, which ranges from a very immature type of love to a diseased form of love. In infatuation one only falls in love—whereas in mature experience one grows into love. In infatuation each person often finds the other meeting some immature or warped emotional need.

Fortunately, infatuation is often self-limiting. Dr. Joyce Brothers feels that the condition usually does not extend beyond two months in time. Possibly not all you readers will agree with this, but it does offer encouragement.

For the Christian, infatuation can prove especially harmful if individuals lose their interest in religious things and in the duties of life. Such persons may spend late hours in courting and have a low concern for morality and religion. (See *Messages to Young People*, pp. 457-459.)

Perhaps I should quickly add that all attraction in the early teen years is not infatuation. Christian teen-agers can maintain a fine and deep relationship that demonstrates a cleanness and unselfish commitment which can surpass many of the relationships entered upon by older persons.

Naturally, all love should be charged with romance (see the Song of Solomon, for example), but should not become top-heavy with it, to the exclusion of all other features that one should consider in selecting a mate. Unfortunately, it is easy to overemphasize romance, especially in our American dating system. The air itself is almost charged with a sick type of romanticism that often becomes a sentimental, sick, and gooey excuse for sex and is the main pressure to marry.

Apply the principles of *Messages to Young People* in your life. It will provide you with a protective code in which to operate. If you follow Mrs. White's advice you will have an insurance policy against a rash and ill-advised affair or marriage.

Fantasies

Some adolescent girls are tempted by fantasies of being molested or raped. Such fantasizing can be an indirect way of removing the guilt of wondering what intercourse is like and of unconsciously wishing for the experience. Having sex forced on them in the fantasy takes away the young woman's responsibility for the act. She is an "innocent victim." Frequent fantasies of this nature would probably indicate an emotional problem in the area of sex.

Fellows sometimes daydream about seducing a woman by

their charm or their powerful masculine appeal or sometimes just by brute force. Such fantasies are only one step removed from the real-life lustful look and desire that Jesus warned against when He expanded the meaning of adultery in Matthew 5:28.

One way to judge your fantasies: If what you daydream about would be wrong in real life, then it is wrong to fantasize about it.

Finding a Future Mate: Reasonable Ideals

Although you should choose your future mate with care, don't set your ideals impossibly high. Keep in mind that you are not likely to find the perfect man or woman. Robert Schumann, the composer, said with wry humor: "When I was a young man I vowed never to marry until I found the ideal woman. Well, I found her—but, alas, she was waiting for the ideal man."

Occasionally, young people set their ideals so high that no one can possibly qualify. As a result these individuals have a good excuse for not marrying—which is most likely the conscious or unconscious reason they have established impossible requirements. It gives them an out. At the same time it makes them appear to have tastes far beyond those of their friends and acquaintances, who settle for lesser mortals.

Jealousy

When you were little, you probably crawled into bed with both of your parents on some mornings and immediately pushed your same-sex parent away. That's a very normal feeling youngsters have, and by now you've long since forgotten about it. You realized gradually that your dad and your mother were special to each other and that no one, even you, could come between them. It was just another step in your emotional and sexual development and in your growth as a person.

Genuine jealousy is another matter. If you suffer from frequent attacks of jealousy, you often feel uncomfortable and unhappy. Most often, in my opinion, this emotion springs from a sense of insecurity that makes some people and some situations a threat to one's peace of mind or emotional happiness.

Whether or not we feel threatened or insecure usually depends on how much attention a particular person is giving us. Any possible competitor who has a seeming advantage over us can make us afraid of losing the special place we have in the loved person's affections. The less jealous we think ourselves to be, the greater is the chance of succumbing to jealousy. An active imagination makes the situation even more painful.

If you wrestle with strong feelings of jealousy, I suggest you talk this over with a counselor you like or some older person whom you trust—this can even be one of your parents! A perceptive adviser can help you dig down inside to see how you look at yourself. A counselor can probably assist you in seeing some of your strong points that you have overlooked or ways of improving yourself that you can quickly make use of.

Jealousy has destroyed many marriages. Get to the root of the problem while you're young so that it won't destroy that which you cherish most later in life.

Acne

As you move through adolescence you may break out with acne. Surely all of you know what I'm talking about. Either you or some friends of yours have had to fight it. One dermatologist has called acne mankind's most common disease.

Blackheads will become a worry. Sometimes they may develop into pustules. Usually the face is the main part of the body affected—the one you least want to be involved. Acne also can spread over the neck and shoulders. Young women may have more trouble with acne before or during menstrual periods. Stress seems to aggravate the condition also.

Sometimes individuals with acne think they have acquired the condition because they have failed to wash thoroughly or have eaten too many sweets and fried foods. However, the main cause of acne is the increased quantity of androgen hormone, which increases the size and the activity of the "fat" glands. Since sweating can make acne worse, you may want to see whether certain kinds of exercise increase the problem.

You may want to see a dermatologist if you have acne. He will recommend a helpful regimen that will control your condition. He will probably tell you to drink at least eight glasses of water a day and to match that with eight hours of sleep. Don't try to "operate" on your pustules—you'll probably make the acne worse.

The good news about acne is that a dermatologist can help alleviate the condition and that you will outgrow this embarrassing plague.

You and Your Parents

Do you fellows remember when you first showered with your dad? Do you young ladies recall the time you bathed with your mother? The size of your dad's sex organs—especially since they were pretty close to eye level—really impressed you fellows! And the size and beauty of your mother's breasts looked pretty impressive to a little girl. You wondered whether you would ever reach that same level of growth. Well, by now you either have or are well on the way.

Sometimes parents feel too embarrassed to talk about the subject of sex comfortably with you. But don't be too hard on them. Most of them grew up feeling that the subject was not nice. Some may even assume that if they talk about sex, you might want to go out and experiment. So reach out to your parents, and let them reach out to you. It's a good sign that you're reading a book like this. And if your folks bought it for you, you now have a bridge on which you can meet to share ideas and feelings in this important area of your growth and development.

Most young people your age long for more independence. Fair enough. But as you break away from those parental ties, do so gently. Respect your parents and all they have done. Recognize the burdens resting on them: worries about having money enough to run the home and to meet your needs, worries about your salvation, worries about your getting sick or hurt, worries about not being good-enough parents . . .

Down deep your parents recognize your right to freedom of choice, even though they wish with all their hearts that you will choose to serve God as they do. But they need to get used to letting go too. As you achieve independence you don't have to fight them and their religious principles just to prove your independence. That's a matter between you and God. Don't run with a crowd without checking to see where they are and where they are heading. "Everybody's doing it" affords no excuse for misconduct when you're a Christian. Christians operate not from majorities, but from principles. Besides, it is rarely true that everyone does it.

Forgive your parents when they lose their tempers or act unreasonable or seem unfair at times. They are sinners in need of grace and growth in the Christian life. Despite their temptations and failures, they do love the Lord—and you. Give them credit, at least, for that.

Remember, apart from striving to be in the kingdom and doing their part in spreading the gospel, they want (if the Lord doesn't come soon) to stay well and to retire comfortably at 65 or thereabouts. They also want to see you mature into adulthood, gain some kind of job competence, remain in good health, stay out of trouble with the law, avoid sexual involvements, and find a good partner for marriage—one they can love and be loved by. They probably look forward to enjoying your children and seeing them well started before they go into the last sleep.

By all means, if you are angry at your folks, don't punish them by having friendships with the kind of people they would not want to have in their home or to include as part of their family. Ultimately you'd only be punishing yourself.

Don't confuse love with sympathy for the underdog or for the social misfit. Don't try to reform someone just by your own love. If someone begins to look attractive to you who has had an unattractive past (wild life, trouble with the law, drugs, divorce), be sure that the individual has learned and changed and is now a mature Christian. You don't want your caring to grow to the point where it would become hard to control. Under these circumstances, pray more than you ever have in your life, and not just formally. Solicit advice from your parents, brothers and sisters, and sensible friends.

"Parents are entitled to a degree of love and respect which is due to no other person. God Himself, who has placed upon them a responsibility for the souls committed to their charge, has ordained that during the earlier years of life, parents shall stand in the place of God to their children. And he who rejects the rightful authority of his parents is rejecting the authority of

God. The fifth commandment requires children not only to yield respect, submission, and obedience to their parents, but also to give them love and tenderness, to lighten their cares, to guard their reputation, and to succor and comfort them in old age. It also enjoins respect for ministers and rulers and for all others to whom God had delegated authority."—*Patriarchs and Prophets*, p. 308.

Purity

Christians cannot enjoy a healthy spiritual life if non-Christian ideas color their thinking about and behavior in sex. The path the Christian travels puts him on a collision course with much of the world's thinking and practice. You have to make a choice—you can't run with the hares and with the hounds at the same time.

The adjectives *pure, chaste,* and *modest* describe the life style Christians choose. They do not regard virginity as a rigid requirement only for plastic people. Christians avoid masturbation, pornography, and company that might expose them to pressure toward unwholesome and unholy thinking or conduct.

During the latter part of the past century, some people took part in a Purity Movement. Men and women, boys and girls, signed purity pledges, each with the heading "Thou God Seest Me."

The men's pledge read like this:

"I hereby solemnly promise by the help of God—

"I. To obey the law of purity in thought and act.

"II. To refrain from, and to discountenance in others, vulgarity of speech and indecent jests and allusions.

"III. To avoid all books, amusement, and associations calculated to excite impure thoughts.

"IV. To uphold the same standard of purity for men and women.

"V. To oppose all laws and customs which tend to the degradation of women and to labor for their reform.

"VI. To endeavor to spread the knowledge of these principles and to aid others in obeying them."

The form for the women read pretty much the same.

"I hereby solemnly promise by the help of God—

"I. To obey the law of purity in thought and act.

"II. To refrain from and to discountenance in others all conversation upon impure subjects, and to avoid all books, amusements, and associations that tend in the direction of impurity.

"III. To be modest in language, behavior, and dress.

"IV. To uphold the same standard of purity for men and women.

"V. To oppose all laws and customs which tend to the degradation of women and to labor for their reform.

"VI. To endeavor to spread the knowledge of these principles and to aid others in obeying them."

Perhaps we should revive this movement and formulate a similar pledge to fit the conditions of our time.

Chapter 9

The Seamy Side of Sex

Before Adam and Eve ate from the forbidden tree, they knew only that which is good. After eating the fruit from that tree, they began learning about an infinite amount of evil. The history of mankind certainly makes that evident.

The entrance of sin stained every phase of life. As rapidly and as destructively as possible the devil tried to turn every attribute of man into the opposite of what God had intended. The sexual part of human nature, one of God's most magnificent and exciting gifts, Satan relentlessly attacked. Humans began indulging their sexuality in ways that hurt and corrupted. Sex became the polluted spring for a wide-flowing stream of pain, heartache, disease, cruelty, and perverted behavior.

Since we live in a world that long ago left the purity of Eden, there are several things on the dark side of sex that we have to know something about—molestation, masturbation, homosexuality, and venereal disease. As in all areas of life, there are rights and wrongs here that young Christians must be aware of.

Molestation

This is a distasteful subject to write about. However, I would be less than frank and honest to write a book about sex education without including some discussion of molestation.

One out of four girls, on the average, will suffer from some form of molestation by the end of adolescence. Most often this will be in the form of the emotional upset and shock that comes from seeing a man exhibiting his genitals. Most likely such an experience will occur near a school or a playground where groups of girls are present. For boys the great majority of contacts come from homosexuals or heterosexuals who have not grown up or have grown up with a kink in their development.

Frederic Storaska, in *How to Say No to a Rapist and Survive,* writes: "It's almost certain that at least once in your life you will be the victim of a 'minor' sexual annoyance . . . such as an obscene phone call, frottage, an exhibitionist, and a Peeping Tom."—Chapter 12. (Frottage means that a man gets sexual stimulation by rubbing against a girl's body, as is possible in a crowded elevator or railroad car.)

Most molesters are men, but fortunately they rarely use physical force or endanger the life of the victim. Usually the molester is an acquaintance or even a family member. Molesters often threaten the young person involved not to tell, or they bribe the youngster with some gift or favor.

A molester usually takes up such behavior because he is not emotionally mature enough to deal with a girl or woman on a normal plane. He gets a charge from his deviant behavior, which makes him feel more like a man (in his twisted interpretation of sexuality). The shock and fear that his action generates increases his excitement.

If you are unfortunate enough to fall victim to such an approach, the good sex education you have received from your parents should help you throw the experience off with a minimum of emotional damage. I hope you can talk it over quickly and easily with them—but never tell the molester that you plan to do this.

If this kind of experience involves a brother, grandfather, uncle, or cousin (and it sometimes does), be sure to talk to your parents about it. If, God forbid, the molester should be your father, you will need to talk things over with your mother. If she doesn't believe you or seems unable to face up to the problem, you can talk with someone whom you deeply trust and respect—a teacher or your pastor. Confide in someone who can help you without breaking your confidence. Remember that sexual overtures from such relatives do not manifest love. They merely intend to use you for the gratification of their sinful and emotionally sick desires.

Most larger communities—and some smaller ones—offer services to help victims of rape or molestation. The staff members in such organizations are trained to understand what has happened and to give all the support needed. They can also help a boyfriend understand why such things happen and show him how he can offer the greatest support for the victim.

In passing here are a few suggestions for your protection:

1. When you go anywhere at night, be sure to have your father or brother as escort (unless you know for sure that everything is absolutely OK). When you have a date with a fellow, be certain that he is dependable and trustworthy and that he will not knowingly take you to places where there is a risk of attack.

2. Avoid blind dates. Accept one (if you don't mind this type of date) only when it includes another couple who are reliable friends and who share your high standards.

3. Don't dress provocatively. Yet it should be kept in mind that rape is often primarily an act of hostility to women, rather than an uncontrollable urge for sex. This is particularly evident when the victim is in her sixties or seventies.

4. Don't park in secluded places and in lovers' lanes. Places young people favor as "parking" spots are naturally the first places that a rapist on the prowl will head for.

5. Don't take for granted that school or hospital grounds are "safe."

6. If you must walk alone at night, stay in well-lighted areas as much as possible.

7. When you are walking alone, stride confidently, directly, and steadily.

8. Walk on the side of the street facing traffic.

9. Avoid walking close to doorways, bushes, and alleys where a rapist might hide.

10. Remain alert when people stop and ask you for directions—never get too close to the car.

11. If danger appears imminent don't hesitate to scream and run.

12. If you are in trouble scream for help or yell, "Fire!"

13. If a stranger offers you a ride accept it only if you will be riding with a woman or an older couple—never accept a ride from a lone man or a boisterous group.

14. Lock all the car doors at *all* times.

15. Park your car only in well-lighted areas.

16. Check the back seat of a parked car before you get inside.

17. Drive to a public place or a police station if you think someone is following you.

18. If your vehicle breaks down open the hood and attach a white cloth to the antenna. Stay inside the locked car if someone stops to help and ask him to call the police or a garage.

Masturbation

Most young people are concerned about the subject of masturbation, so that makes it important enough to speak about. It seems as though masturbation can tempt an individual all through life, but particularly during the early years.

Some people don't know how to define masturbation, so I shall be specific. A young man masturbates when he manipulates his penis by hand to the point of ejaculating. A young woman masturbates by stimulating her clitoris by hand or with some object to the point of orgasm.

Ellen White has quite a bit to say about self-abuse, or secret vice, which most of us recognize as older names for masturbation. The three-volume *Index* to her writings has several columns of references under the heading "Secret vice." If your home library does not have the *Index* but has a set of the *Testimonies*—and I hope it does—you can find a great deal of counsel about masturbation in the second volume. Check in its index under "Vice, secret." If you attend one of our church schools or academies, you will find these books in its library.

Mrs. White states that she received special revelations about the prevalence of this habit in the families of church members. She saw that many children had taken up the practice of masturbation.

In the book *Child Guidance,* a compilation of material from her pen, she tells of a middle-aged man who practiced this habit. He had taken very ill, and friends had asked her and her husband to pray for him. Since they were just visiting his church, they did not know the man, so did not feel free to pray for him. However, they presented their quandary to the Lord in their evening prayer. In a dream that night the Lord told Mrs. White that they should not pray for the sick man. God would not accept a prayer in his behalf. Why? This man had been practicing masturbation from his early years—and still persisted in doing it. She adds the sad comment about another man practicing this vice that he died a self-murderer. She observed that the purity of heaven will not be marred by his presence.

In her account Ellen White uses the word *abomination*. She doubtless borrowed the term from Leviticus 18, where it describes adultery, homosexuality, incest, and bestiality (having intercourse with an animal).

Mrs. White elsewhere plainly warns that young people "cannot be Christians unless they entirely cease to practice this hellish, soul-and-body-destroying vice" (*Testimonies*, vol. 2, p. 410). She states that "when persons are addicted to the habit of self-abuse, it is impossible to arouse their moral sensibilities to appreciate eternal things or to delight in spiritual exercises" (*ibid.*, p. 470).

Mrs. White also insists that the habit affects many organs of the body and even causes disease. She writes that it interferes with the best functioning of the brain and nervous system and damages one's personality.

I have to admit, in all honesty, that at the present time the fields of medicine and psychology have provided practically no evidence to back up her statements about the damage masturbation does to the body. However, in my former book, *God Invented Sex*, and in the book on sex education written for your parents, I call attention to the vindication modern science has provided for her writings.

"As a people we point out how reliable and trustworthy her counsel was and is, especially when she saw ahead to discoveries only recently made. Time after time we have seen her statements vindicated, even when out of harmony with the medical and psychological opinion of her day. They include the relationship between faulty diet and juvenile delinquency, the beneficial effect of sunlight, dangers in the excessive use of salt, the presence of animal fats and sugar in helping to produce blood-vessel diseases, the value of walking as an exercise, the dangers of hypnosis as a 'mind cure,' risks in misuse of X-ray, the tremendous importance of psychosomatic medicine, the relation between stress and longevity, the power of prenatal influence, the statement that 'germs' are a causative factor in cancer, the destructive power of tobacco, and the relation between drugs and birth defects."—Page 164.

Then I end on this note: "If we think she is wrong about masturbation, we had better reexamine our understanding of the operation of prophecy in the church. If we feel she is right, we need to act on what she wrote, pending eventual confirmation."—*Ibid.*

If you determine to heed her advice, you can enter God's presence at any time and ask for the power of His Spirit to help you refrain from masturbation. In view of all the stimulation that faces young people today and the general easygoing attitude toward masturbation, you will need His continuing support in controlling your sex drive so that you do not resort to masturbation.

Remember, no sexual sin is the unpardonable sin. The same Lord who told us to forgive our brother seventy times can hardly do any less Himself. If you wish to seek forgiveness for masturbating, rest assured that God will gladly provide it.

In my opinion, to live a clean life sexually—in thought and act—during the teen years is one of the most persuasive arguments in favor of the power of Christianity. It probably provides the hardest test of Christian commitment and consecration. Yet there are young people who exemplify these standards.

Suggestions for Dealing With Masturbation

1. Decide whether or not Ellen White has spoken for the Lord when she mentions the possible serious consequences of masturbation. Then take her warnings to heart and ask Him to help you achieve and maintain mastery over this habit.

2. Recognize that in the adolescent years, as you develop sexually and yet remain years away from the possibility of marriage, the habit can strongly appeal to you as a way to relieve sexual tension. These tensions—in both young men and women—are often "drained away" by dreams or sexual arousal during sleep. Fellows have a particular form of release—wet dreams, or nocturnal emissions, already referred to.

3. Also recognize that the world around you will not make

your determination easy to follow.

a. Most people tend to accept masturbation as a necessary part of human sexual development. Exceptions are the Roman Catholic Church, the Orthodox Jews, and some evangelical faiths.

b. Most of the fellows and some of the girls in your nonchurch social and school groups will engage in this habit with fair regularity.

c. Your world presents endless sexual stimulation from TV, music, some books, and many conversations. Magazines often publish special articles on the subject.

d. Some fellows buy sex magazines and masturbate while they imagine they are having intercourse with the nude women in the pictures. Young women may "reverse" this imagery, fantasizing themselves as being overcome by a lover.

The body and mind can experience emotions as though the acts were really being carried out. Dr. John Berecz, of Andrews University, has said: "Daydreams, fantasies, mental images, are real. When you vividly imagine doing something, your brain fires many of the same neural circuits that would be fired if you were actually doing the behavior. . . . Imagined behavior is real behavior."

Ellen White said the same thing, but not with Dr. Berecz's scientific words: "Exciting love stories and impure pictures have a corrupting influence. Novels are eagerly perused by many, and, as a result, their imagination becomes defiled. . . . The heart is corrupted through the imagination. The mind takes pleasure in contemplating scenes which awaken the lower and baser passions. These vile images, seen through defiled imagination, corrupt the morals and prepare the deluded, infatuated beings to give loose rein to lustful passions."—*Testimonies*, vol. 2, p. 410.

4. Some young people learn the habit during an overnight visit in another fellow's or girl's home. That's why Ellen White did not permit her children to make visits of this kind and discouraged children of other families from staying at her home overnight.

5. Since you regard the Lord as the Creator who designed your sex organs, you will accept from Him any advice that He

offers for the healthy use of these organs.

6. Since the Lord loved you enough to die for you, you will cheerfully put yourself under His loving authority.

7. Especially guard against masturbation when you feel left out by any group, or when you think that there's nothing to do and nowhere to go, or when you feel down.

8. You can't control the tendency to masturbate by concentrating all your energy on trying not to masturbate. That's like my telling you not to think of a black cat for the next ten minutes. You are tempted to think of a black cat in order not to think of a black cat! When the temptation to masturbate floods over you, fill your mind with other thoughts or immediately switch to some activity that will occupy your attention. Just before going to sleep can be a tough time.

9. If you do slip into the practice, don't try to atone for it by making rash promises or lifetime resolutions. Such an approach usually is self-defeating. Instead let your resistance build up by making Jesus the center of your life. Let Him answer the door when the evil one knocks on the door of your heart.

10. Don't stop masturbating just to avoid the consequences. Fear is a poor motivation. Let your motive be positive—you desire to please the Lord by directing your sexual life according to His counsel.

11. Remember that masturbation, although a serious habit, is not the only measure of a man or woman. Don't let your struggle with masturbation fill your whole world and become the only measure of your standing with God.

Homosexuality

Most of you have doubtless encountered such words as *queer, fairy, faggot,* and *gay*—common terms for the male homosexual. Probably the most common word for female homosexuals is *lesbian*.

The male's way of having sex with another male is summed up in the words of one homosexual author: "For gay men there are three erotic zones—mouth, penis, and anus." For the female a comparable list might include: hands, breast, clitoris, and vagina.

Heterosexuals (those who make love to members of the

opposite sex) find it difficult to understand why or how these people prefer to make love to members of their own sex. Maybe you wonder what makes a person homosexual. Well, professionals who work in the field of sex can't agree on any single cause. Some who work in the field of sex still think that parents have a lot to do with a young person's becoming a homosexual. They suggest that a hostile father who has little to do with his son or who is a weak and ineffectual male figure can provide a possible starting point for male homosexuality. The mother may then get too close (psychologically) to the son, tying him to her with strong emotional cords. She may favor him with more attention than is normal in the mother-son relationship. She may sometimes be even closer to him than to his father.

Some studies of the mothers of lesbians report them as being critical of their daughters and preventing them from engaging in normal feminine activities in the home. These mothers have tended to defeminize their daughters and have often interfered with the development of normal relationships with males. The fathers of lesbians have supposedly not provided suitable male models for their daughters. They often dominate and get too close (emotionally) to the girls. They seem to compete with their daughters' boyfriends. They cherish strict but unhealthy views of sex, and they prevent the development of normal sex maturity in their daughters.

On the other hand, one of the psychiatrists at Loma Linda University, Dr. Ray B. Evans, suggests that the evidence indicates that the fathers and mothers of homosexuals have had as good relations with their children as have parents of heterosexuals.

Dr. Evans' perspective has been substantiated by a ten-year study conducted at the Kinsey Institute and published in the fall of 1981. After interviewing 1,500 men and women (both heterosexual and homosexual), the researchers concluded that parents have almost no influence over their child's developing sexual preference.

Dr. Wardell Pomeroy, a top authority on sex, thinks that environmental factors can influence children in that direction. He agrees that parents have only limited control over the way their children turn out sexually.

Other authorities regard homosexuality as a way of getting stuck in an immature kind of sexual development. Some interpret it as a case of wrong development. Others consider it a deep-rooted personality disorder.

You have no doubt concluded that all these suggestions simply add to the confusion as to what really brings on homosexuality. You are probably right. Homosexuality remains a mystery.

You may assume that you can easily spot a homosexual. But nine out of ten homosexuals do not look or act like the stereotype. The fellows who are swishy or who dress in drag (as women) can be easily spotted, of course. One young homosexual told me candidly that he was working on his wrist action and his walk. He wanted to stay "in the closet" and avoid drawing attention to himself. (Today more and more homosexuals frankly make known their sexual preference.)

Some people feel that all homosexuals dislike those of the opposite sex. This is not true. Homosexuals often enjoy having special occasions with those of the other gender. Others feel that all homosexuals are likely to tempt young people into their way of life. This also is false. (What about those heterosexuals who seduce or molest girls?)

However, one recent case in my own State of North Carolina, reported in the Charlotte *Observer*, points up the need for alertness on the part of you young people and your parents. A coach whom boys greatly admired was accused of engaging in sexual acts with twenty-seven boys. He had never been seen having dates with women and he always had some fellows around him. He paid particular attention to blond boys between 9 and 14. He gave them gifts or money. He even took some to church services. After he got them to have sex with him he would indicate that it would be a sin to tell anyone about their encounter. Within a period of three to four months he had been involved in sixty-two contacts.

At first it was very difficult ("like pulling teeth," the reporter wrote) to get the boys to talk about what had happened. You can understand, too, that the parents, when they found out about it, did not want to go to court and testify. They didn't want their boys to be called homosexuals and damaged emotionally. Later, fortunately, they changed their minds and decided to prosecute.

In fairness I should state that such conduct on the part of an adult homosexual is quite uncommon. It probably occurs much less frequently, relatively speaking, than does the molestation of girls by heterosexuals. But you should be on guard against such approaches, no matter who the man is or how much adults respect him.

If a fellow has had some sort of sex play with another fellow, or a girl with another girl, this does not necessarily mean that they are on the road to homosexuality. (I refer here to a few occasions—not a continuing preference for this type of behavior.)

Likewise, if you fellows in your early years of adolescence develop a strong liking for an older fellow, or if you girls worship an older woman, this does not mean that you have homosexual tendencies. Most young people go through a period of crushes.

Perhaps—if you are a fellow—you do not feel like being quite as rough and tough as some of the other fellows in your crowd. Don't worry. That doesn't mean there's something wrong with your sexual orientation.

Sometimes a young man can worry about being homosexual just because he is not doing too well with life in general. As Dr. S. M. Woods, director of Student Psychiatric Services in the University of Southern California at Los Angeles, puts it, the chain of thinking and feeling (often unconscious) runs like this: "I am a failure. . . . I am castrated. . . . I am not a man. . . . I'm like a woman. . . . I am a homosexual."

If somehow you begin to worry a bit about your sexual development, talk over your concerns with some older person who is competent to help you, whom you like and respect, and who can keep confidences. You can be sure he won't look down on you. He'll be glad to help you through your valley of the shadows.

As you would guess, the homosexuals' way of having sex leads to venereal diseases in parts of the body other than the usual genital areas—for example, the throat, the anus, and the rectum. Since they often are more sexually promiscuous than heterosexuals, their rate of venereal diseases is comparatively higher, particularly in diseases of the rectum and anus.

Over the years there will probably be—perhaps already are—homosexuals in your social world. You should be sure enough in your heterosexuality that you are not in any way vulnerable to any overtures for homosexual sex.

We should differentiate between persons who are practicing homosexuals and those who have that kind of orientation but who do not engage in homosexual sex. Certainly the second type deserve special honor, since they must fight against odds that heterosexuals never have to meet. Even the places these individuals live in can be centers of temptation—camps, residence halls, et cetera.

The main problem for Christians is how to classify homosexuality. Is it all sin, all sickness, a mixture of both, or just a different way of living? Naturally, homosexuals don't like to be classified as sick. Many feel that they have as much right to be what they are as do heterosexuals.

The Scriptures, as you probably know, condemn the practice without qualification (for example, see Gen. 19:1-25; Lev. 18:22; Judges 19, 20; Rom. 1:26-32; 1 Cor. 6:9, 10).

And although we must condemn homosexuality as contrary to the will and wish of God, we must recognize that some homosexuals have grown into this type of sexual orientation without having actively chosen such a way of life.

Anyone suffering painful anxiety and serious perplexity about his or her sexual orientation may want to contact Quest Learning Center, Route 1, Box 224, Reading, Pennsylvania 19607. This organization is dedicated to helping those with homosexual tendencies—particularly Seventh-day Adventists. It has received the support of the General Conference because its philosophy and approach harmonize with the position the denomination took at the 1981 Spring Meeting. A list of competent counselors to whom persons can be referred is available to Adventist church pastors.

The report in the May 21, 1981, issue of the *Adventist Review* stated: "The church must extend compassion and understanding to homosexuals seeking Christ's deliverance, restoration, and redemptive grace. It must show concern by making every effort to develop a ministry that will meet their particular needs. It is not possible for the church to condone practicing homosexuality, nor is it possible to grant 'equal rights' to such individuals within the church. The efforts of the church must be focused on individuals, rather than on groups, who desire help and deliverance. The church finds it impossible to endorse organizations or individuals (1) who contend that homosexuality be considered an acceptable alternative, (2) who are satisfied with being homosexuals, and (3) who resist or reject change. The church cannot negotiate with organized groups who refer to themselves as SDA gays or lesbians, nor can it establish 'diplomatic relations' with such groups when doing so might be considered recognition and official endorsement of a deviant philosophy and life style.''

Venereal Diseases

This kind of trouble should never become a factor in the life of a Christian. However, sometimes Christians may stray off the road and get involved with persons of loose morals. It is not uncommon to pick up some type of sexually transmitted disease (STD) through intimate sexual contacts with such individuals. (Today the term *sexually transmitted diseases* is replacing the older *venereal diseases.*)

Estimates suggest that 2.5 million teen-agers contract an STD every year. The incidence of these diseases among those ranging from age 12 to 20 is three times that of the remaining adult population. Today's sexual freedom probably is the main reason for the amazing spread of these diseases. One authority has observed that some teen-agers seem to consider STD ''a badge of honor.'' Between sixty-five thousand and one hundred thousand young women become permanently sterile each year in the United States because of pelvic gonorrhea.

Statistics, of course, are based on reported cases and estimates derived from those figures. As you can easily guess, the public health authorities never know the actual number of cases in any given community.

Male homosexuals, compared with heterosexuals, lead a very active sex life. A survey of college-age homosexuals found that they had eight times the number of partners that heterosexuals had. Some male homosexuals encounter a thousand or more partners in a lifetime. As a result, the rate of sexually transmitted diseases is comparatively higher among homosexuals than among heterosexuals.

Incidentally, a problem that often accompanies STD is the chance of acquiring body and pubic lice. A physician can prescribe medication that will eradicate these unwelcome guests. Over-the-counter medications are not effective.

Genital herpes—Genital herpes, wrongly called the disease of love (more honest name: disease of copulation), is one of the most common STDs in America. Each year five hundred thousand people contract the disease. It travels from mouth, penis, and anus to similar, or analogous, organs in the partner.

Usually symptoms appear from two to eight days after infection. Men develop painful blisters on the penis. Women may find them at the entrance to the vagina, but more likely the blisters "hide" in the organs or on the cervix.

If a pregnant mother has an active herpes infection either on the cervix or on the lips at the entrance to the vagina at the time of delivery, it can cause the death of the baby or one or more of several severe complications, including blindness. Delivery, in such a case, should be by Caesarean section.

Even without treatment the symptoms disappear in from one to four weeks. However, the viruses merely go underground, usually lurking in the lower spine area. It seems that the viruses can reside here as long as the host lives. Symptoms can reappear when the body conditions stimulate them. Treatment can help, but as of the time of writing there was no known cure for the disease, although some quack medications have been palmed off on the unsuspecting public. Researchers are working hard at finding a cure. Perhaps by now they have found one. Check with your physician. (See "The New Scarlet Letter," *Time*, Aug. 2, 1982, pp. 62-66.)

Nongonococcal Urethritis (NGU)—Another sexually transmitted disease is nongonococcal urethritis. It competes with genital herpes as the most common STD in the country. One director of a city department of health says that, despite the increasing incidence of NGU, many physicians hold the opinion that it is a mild, insignificant infection without any serious complications.

Since it is not as painful as gonorrhea, infected men do not go as quickly for treatment. In men it can result in inflammation of the epididymus and sterility. It can inflame the female pelvic organs, causing sterility. It can produce eye infections and pneumonia in very young children. The disease causes a discharge in women and urethrel drips in men. This discharge can range from a clear mucous type to a yellow purulence and may cause a burning sensation during urination in both sexes.

Gonorrhea (drip, the clap)—Gonorrhea is epidemic in scope, with a widespread increase among teen-agers. Eight out of ten women who contract the disease, at least in its early stages, show no noticeable symptoms. A small percentage of men also exhibit no early symptoms. In Los Angeles County alone probably as many as forty-five thousand women do not know that they have gonorrhea and are infecting their sex partners. Another estimate is that one in ten girls between the ages of 15 and 21 has gonorrhea but does not realize it.

The chances of a male catching the infection as a result of one act of intercourse with an infected female are about one in four. If a female has intercourse with an infected male, the possibility of her contracting the infection is practically certain.

Over the years the gonorrhea germs "have learned" how to fight against penicillin. About forty years ago only one hundred thousand units of that antibiotic would ordinarily knock out gonorrhea. Today the dosage has to be close to 5 million units. American troops from the Viet Nam area imported a penicillin-resistant form of gonorrhea into the United States. Since this form does not respond at all to penicillin, physicians must resort to specialized drugs in order to clear the system of the disease.

Symptoms in the male include pus draining or dripping from the penis and a burning sensation two to eight days after infection. A puslike discharge may develop in from three to twenty-one days. Or there may be no symptoms at all.

Gonorrhea frequently spreads to the eyes, mouth and throat, joints, heart, rectum, brain, and skin. Although the infection normally is transmitted by sexual activity, it is possible for the disease to be transmitted by contaminated fingers, rectal thermometers, enema tips, or by sleeping with an infected parent. One of my counselees, for example, innocently contracted gonorrhea at the age of 6. As you might guess, too, it is not rare for a philandering husband to bring the disease home to his unsuspecting wife.

Syphilis—People with syphilis usually develop a chancre, a painless sore, within two to six weeks after infection. Usually the chancre appears on a genital organ, but sometimes it shows up on another part of the body, such as a lip or an eyelid. A sore may remain out of sight in the vagina, also. The chancre is the primary syphilis. It disappears in two to six weeks.

In the secondary stage the spirochetes that cause the disease move to different parts of the body by way of the blood. In six to eight weeks after the sore has healed, the infected individual can manifest an illness that resembles flu. There is a generalized enlargement of the lymph nodes, and usually a rash appears over most of the body, often on the palms and soles. The secondary stage lasts for one to two months, and during this time the disease is highly contagious. Unfortunately, the rash can look like a symptom of practically every skin disease known, so the syphilis may be hard to diagnose. Some hair may fall out.

Once again the spirochetes go underground—this time for a long period of years. This stage is called tertiary syphilis. Eventually the disease can injure any organ, even doing heavy damage to the brain. Because syphilis can be diagnosed by a blood test and can be defeated with antibiotics, most people with the disease never enter the destructive third stage.

Chlamydia—Another STD should be mentioned—chlamydia. One of the most recent reports on this is contained in an interview with Dr. Priscilla Wyrick, a bacteriologist on the staff of the University of North Carolina, as reported in the *Charlotte Observer* of November 2, 1980.

She points out that chlamydia affects three million Americans; that while it does not threaten life, it "is the world's leading cause of preventable blindness and can result in male and female sterility." She states that most people who have it don't have symptoms, and when they do, the disease is diagnosed as gonorrhea. The interview report concludes with this depressing statement: "Because chlamydia—unlike 95% of known bacteria—is able to get inside cells in the body, it remains difficult to cure."

Perhaps you know someone who is worrying about the possibility of having an STD but who is afraid or unable to talk to his parents about it. Suggest that he call the local department of public health and make an appointment to see a doctor. In most States such information is kept confidential. The caller can check on this before making an appointment.

One final warning: These diseases can be picked up in the intimacies of foreplay. One does not need to engage in intercourse to contract a sexually transmitted disease.

Chapter 10

Dating—Bane or Boon?

Sometimes Adventists seem to have a "village mentality" when it comes to dating patterns. A young couple enjoy one or two dates, and the rest of the community assumes they have a commitment to a deeper relationship. Too often we allow little time or leeway for young people to explore each others' tastes, feelings, and ideas. Yet we will spend quite a bit of time shopping around before we purchase a dress, a pair of shoes, a purse, or a car.

From my conversations with young people on Adventist campuses, I have found that they yearn for more opportunities for young men and women to interact without couple-dating as a prerequisite. Our academies and colleges should take the lead in fostering such opportunities and creating a more comfortable, safer, and more promising program for the largest number of students.

Adolescent preferences—including tastes in people—can change in a short time. For this reason no one should feel that the ending of a relationship after a few dates means one of the individuals is undesirable. Until more mature preferences shape themselves, a lot of movement in and out of relationships is desirable. It is hardly likely that, in the first or second time around the circle of acquaintances, one can find the young woman or young man who fits in most comfortably and happily with one's future life.

Many men take a lot of time to pick out a car, which they can dispose of if it does not meet their needs. Choosing a future husband or wife involves deeper considerations than speed, cost of operation, depreciation, et cetera. Now, not every car one chooses not to purchase is inferior. Indeed, a car not selected may be even a sounder buy than the one finally acquired. Girls or fellows, then, whose dates cool off do not have to feel like rejects. They should recognize that there was no deep-down clicking together. Many times breaking off a relationship is an unrecognized blessing.

Cars

In the United States automobiles provide opportunities for dating and set patterns of dating. If properly used they can be a real blessing. Many young men consider the car a symbol of their *machismo*. Some fellows use a car to counterbalance their feelings of inferiority. By showing off in driving, they expose themselves and their dates to danger. Young ladies should avoid dates with such fellows.

Dating is also governed to some degree by the relationship between the young man and his parents as to the privilege of using the family car (or one of them if they have more than one).

For quite a few couples the young man's sense of power behind the wheel creates an extra shot of tension that makes sex seem more exciting in a car than in an ordinary place like home. The car can provide an additional undercurrent of thrill, especially if the couple parks in a romantic spot. Going to sexually explicit drive-in movies can quickly stir up surges of feeling that may easily get out of hand. (We should be able to assume, of course, that young Seventh-day Adventists do not attend the theater, but . . .)

Young adults will not abuse the privilege of having access to an automobile. Instead they will enjoy—but not exploit—the freedom cars can provide. Christian principles should guide relationships regardless of the mode or circumstances of the date.

Going Steady

Sometimes going steady means little more than a convenience arrangement for the time being. Both persons know that they have a partner on call, with no need to wonder or to look around when an interesting event is on the calendar. In such a situation, going steady may not pose any serious problems.

But going steady can have different meanings in different social groups. In some instances it can be almost equal to engagement. Then teen-agers assume that they have found the "right" person. However, at such an age and with limited chances of meeting a wide variety of other young people, how can a teen-ager be sure that this person is the best for him or for her?

Young people need to recognize that there are quite a few suitable persons in the world, any one of whom they could marry happily. Teens don't need to decide too quickly that they have met the one and only, because there really is no such person.

In fact, sometimes when a couple are going steady, a very attractive new young person enters the neighborhood or school, or joins the church. Suddenly you may wish that you are not already mortgaged by the steady arrangement. Rest assured that your friends will tell the newcomer that you are already taken. This, of course, narrows the field and increases their chances of dating the new person.

Occasionally a couple feel so committed to each other after a long series of dates that they do not dare to break up. They have become a habit to each other, and they hope that when they marry they will experience the kind of love such a union requires.

The closeness of going steady can cause biology to take over more quickly and strongly than it should. In fact, going steady may produce a false sense of intimacy simply because no one else is eligible to dilute the amount of exposure a person has to just one individual.

Many parents feel that they should discourage their teens from going steady. Some feel it can be accepted if the couple keep the relationship healthy. By healthy they usually mean that the couple know what is right and practice it and that they realize getting serious too early would be—to use a modern term—counterproductive.

Parents and Rules

Your parents should have an understanding with you

regarding the time you should return home from a date. The curfew can vary with your age.

A curfew set by fair and concerned parents demonstrates their love. We try to protect those we care for, and the curfew puts a fence around a youngster's reputation and, sometimes, provides a necessary margin of safety. Parents who let their children do whatever they want are not really loving parents. They have abdicated the responsibility that goes with parenthood.

It should be taken for granted that you will not go to parties at which the participants drink or dance. Young men should know that a date does not include "parking" privileges.

Also, your parents will feel a lot better if they know the car used on your date is in good condition. I remember one time when my younger daughter went on a date with a young man who had borrowed a car for the evening. When she had not returned home by three in the morning, the muscles in my lower back began to ache. I had visions of a wreck, with no car coming by to help. When they arrived home the young man admitted sheepishly that they had had two flat tires within an hour in places where he couldn't get any help. As for me, I had aged a few weeks in a few hours!

Young Ladies Set Limits

Without becoming paranoid, remember that young men may have sex on their minds on any or all dates. Some will actually consider dating as a campaign, long or short, in which they must make the proper moves to reach their goal. They may plead love. They may describe the sexual tension that wracks their bodies, brought on by your power to arouse a consuming hunger in a man. They may urge you to be "normal" and do what everyone else does.

Whatever approach is made, you have the right from the first date (if there are any more) to set limits that make it possible for you to enjoy the type of relationship you feel measures up to your Christian standards and your own personal tastes and hopes.

A Christian young man, while he recognizes the reality of sex and its power, will join you in maintaining behavior that does not encourage a lapse from high ideals. He will agree with you that engaging in premarital sex is premature and selfish. It focuses too heavily on the physical element in the relationship.

Self-respect plays an important part when it comes to postponing sex until marriage. The more Christian young people recognize their value in the Lord's eyes, the more comfortable they can be with their decision to remain chaste. The more they see their own worth as a person, the less vulnerable they will be to the temptation of premarital sex. The young women will feel secure in the face of the charge that they are neurotic, frigid, and hung up. And the young men will realize that the loss of their own virginity does not constitute manhood.

Love and Reality

Most young ladies of academy and high school age begin dating at a younger age than do the fellows. A young woman in her early teens will most likely show interest in young men in their middle or late teens, because older fellows are usually more at ease socially and can match the young lady's more advanced social consciousness.

However, the early-teen fellow has probably already experienced some orgasms, whereas the teen-age girl probably has not. Eight out of ten boys in the general population have by the age of 14 experienced wet dreams and/or masturbation. The average girl will usually lag behind him in this type of experience.

Group dating should be the usual practice during early teens. As you move into the middle teens you will be more ready for couple dating, or twosomes. Double dating with a couple who share your high standards can help shield you from the emotional and biological pressures that single dating can sometimes encourage.

Normal dating can build up your self-confidence by making you feel popular and attractive. But if you don't feel like dating for the time being, don't let the crowd around you stampede you into it. You have every right to be yourself and to set your own pace on how and when you move toward the opposite sex. Some young persons prefer to grow up within themselves more before they reach out to others in the same process of growth.

As you would expect, during the teen years the word *love* takes on newer and deeper meanings, but it usually has not yet matured to the stage really needed for the lifelong commitment of marriage. You see, no one has discovered a way to convert love into furniture, food, medical assistance, tuition, and clothing without working for them. (I am aware that some people get money and things as gifts and that some steal them from other people.) And financial pressures have ruined many otherwise promising marriages. No young man has the right to ask a woman to marry him unless he either can support a wife or is involved in an education and/or work plan that promises this kind of competence by the time of the proposed wedding date.

A couple can also reckon on the wife's earning potential as a part of the future income. But her part must be balanced by the possibility of childbirth and the impact children will have on the family budget. A couple who want babies should try to figure out the financial ramifications when the mother has to stop working so she can have the baby, and whether she will return to work in a short time or wait until the child enters first grade.

Of course, if both partners do not wish to have children and are sure that they will adopt a totally safe method of contraception, they can estimate their future in terms of one or both incomes. Before making such a decision, the couple may want to read Mrs. White's description of what can happen to a man and woman in a childless marriage.

Petting and Necking

Necking involves caressing above the neck, mostly kissing. Petting usually refers to all kinds of caressing below the neck and can go to the point of ejaculation and orgasm or stop just short of them, which requires a pretty strong braking system. Fellows should realize that long or frequent periods of petting can cause congestive inflammation of the prostate gland—an uncomfortable condition at best.

Petting often starts out low key enough, but when some young men see barrier after barrier fall they suddenly want to move on to intercourse itself. Caressing of the breasts may be an early step to other gestures. A young man may interpret acceptance of this as tacit permission to go on to more intimate petting. Since the breasts are not as intimate as the vagina and the clitoris, a couple may feel that they have not gone "too far."

Petting can bring on a drive to go "all the way." After all, in marriage it forms a natural part of foreplay. Thus even a fellow who is not a particularly sensitive or skillful lover—and not too many are—can arouse a sexual response in a young woman that surprises her.

Some couples find petting addictive, arousing the desire for stronger doses of intimacy. Then should the couple break up, they will likely feel that they have begun a course of "cold turkey." Sensual appetites once aroused and fed can make quite a physical and emotional burden when they must be neglected.

Petting often poses a great temptation for young women who have a low opinion of their feminine attractiveness. For example, if a young woman considers her breasts to be too small she will likely feel flattered if she discovers that her date finds them attractive. These young women need to remember that a man is aroused not only by attractiveness but also by a willingness to allow him to take the lead in physical intimacy.

Once again the double standard comes into play. Society expects the young woman to set the limits on petting. In one way this makes sense, for she has a great deal more at stake in terms of possible unhappy consequences. (No one has ever seen a pregnant young man—although occasionally a man may experience false pregnancy.) She also faces the possibility of acquiring a lowered reputation in the social and religious world of her family, school, and church—especially if the fellow brags about their conduct.

(Christian couples believe that all their conduct is open to the eyes of the Lord, and they don't want to indulge in any behavior that grieves the unseen Watcher. At the same time they are aware that true love and clean sexual hunger meet with the Lord's complete approval.)

A young woman does not owe a fellow the reward of petting as pay for taking her out. Fellows who expect this are too cheap to consider as potential candidates for more friendship. No young lady has to buy popularity by granting all the favors many other women may grant. Remember that the less of something good, the higher its value: like gold, stamps, or even pistachios.

Keep in mind that I have based this discussion on Christian principles. By way of contrast, some adults argue that petting is a good way for young people to explore and experience their own sexuality and that of others. Some think it offers a necessary preparatory course for the sex life of marriage.

One sex educator has gone so far as to recommend noncoital petting that climaxes in orgasm. In her view this is perfectly safe and perfectly adapted to the needs of young men and young women. They can do it at home and with the knowledge and consent of their parents.

It is probably unrealistic to expect adolescent couples to refrain from all physical contact. Perhaps some forms of caressing, appropriate to the depth of the relationship, are compatible with Christian ideals. However, Christian couples will remember that the apostle John warned against "the lust of the flesh, and the lust of the eyes." It is easy for the attraction between two people to operate on the level of sensual appetite rather than on the plane of responsible loving.

Here's a formula leading up to a happy and lasting marriage:

The young man and the young woman should be as mature as is possible for their age level—and beyond their teens when they marry. They should begin with a friendship that lasts long enough for them to get acquainted with each other and with their families and friends. If their friendship begins growing into love, they move naturally into courtship and later engagement. At all times they will pace themselves and express their affections in proper and acceptable ways. The principles of modesty and purity will govern their lives. They will avoid situations that might tempt them to break through the limits they have set and will save any too-intimate kind of lovemaking for marriage.

Unrealistic? Not at all. Christian couples can, by God's grace, conduct themselves in such an admirable manner.

Drugs

In the days ahead you will face difficulties and problems, disappointments and heartaches. Depression and anxiety will occasionally be your lot. But you can survive these periods by relying on your own physical and emotional strengths if you undergird them with prayer. You want to remain connected with Him who is, after all, the source of all strength and healing of body and mind.

A few of you may need the temporary help of some prescribed drug to carry you through a period when your own resources seem particularly diminished. The Lord sometimes chooses to help us through the judicious use of medications. I see no sin in making use of such aids. We can compare them in a sense to braces or supports or crutches, which we get rid of as quickly as possible. We certainly don't want to become addicted to them.

Some people may require a prescriptive medication to correct an imbalance in their body chemistry. Such drugs serve the purpose of relieving tension, lessening depression, or lessening excessive fatigue or pain.

Choose a physician of your own faith if he or she is available. Such an individual will be more likely to combine medical knowledge with the counsel gained from the Bible and the writings of Mrs. White. Stay away from all drugs that do not serve medical purposes under a doctor's supervision.

Some drugs, stimulants, produce an up feeling—an artificial high. Another type, depressants, help one unwind. By mixing these two types of drugs a person can play a game of emotional seesaw.

Another class of drugs, the hallucinogens, accurately carry the slang label of "mind benders." They can cause a person to see himself and the world around him in an unideal way. They can affect the operations of the mind in a negative manner.

As you move through adolescence you experience quite a few changes in your physical and emotional development. *Why add the disturbing and harmful effects of drugs to this process?* Treat your body with as much care as you have for a pet you love or for the car that you baby.

It should not be necessary to scare you into leaving drugs alone. Your body is a temple of the Holy Spirit. Nothing should enter it that will in any way hurt its intended operation or mar its attractiveness. Instead of fear or caution, let your reason for leaving drugs alone be your deep respect not only for your own mind and body but also for the One who designed you after His image. He sustains your body and mind every second you live.

You have read a lot about drugs and have heard lectures at school about their harmful effects, but perhaps the following items have not come to your attention, especially since they deal with the relation between drugs and sex.

The chances are that in the average school population, from junior high on up, half the students have tried marijuana once. One out of ten high school seniors smokes pot every day.

Marijuana *seems* to have an aphrodisiac effect (arousing sexual desire) because it loosens the emotional controls and makes one feel more artificially alive in this sense. But the fact is that marijuana lowers the production of sperm. (Fellows, note.) It also definitely damages the genes and chromosomes.

Dr. Robert G. Heath, chairman of psychiatry and neurology at Tulane University, has discovered that the ingredient in marijuana which causes the high also destroys brain cells—and no new ones replace the destroyed brain cells. This brain damage, in turn, injures the physical, mental, and emotional health of the pot smoker. Marijuana does not make life better. It merely makes our "glasses" rosy-hued.

Alcohol is another problem drug. It lowers a person's inhibitions. With less moral power an individual finds it much more difficult to control his words and actions. Under the influence of alcohol a person thinks he is an aggressive lover—and perhaps a more inventive one. However, this is a delusion. As one writer puts it, the courage is not up; rather the fears are down.

Alcohol does more than lower the inhibitions and moral restraints. It also reduces the testosterone level in the blood, and testosterone brings on male puberty and controls the male sex drive and ability to have intercourse. (Fellows, note.)

Through the years you have often heard about the damaging effects of smoking on one's health. The advertisements for cigarettes, of course, show virile men in outdoor activities or on tough jobs. They even suggest that men who smoke have a lot more of what it takes to be successful lovers. But smoking cannot make a man more masculine, more healthy, more sexually effective, or, for that matter, more attractive. In fact, the evidence now seems to show that smoking can affect sexual health. Men who suffer from impotence—the inability to have an erection—often improve in their sexual performance once they stop smoking.

You young women need not feel too smug at this point. Overwhelming evidence indicates that smoking poses a high risk for prospective mothers. Smoking increases your chances of having a stillborn child or a baby with low weight at birth, who eats more poorly and gains more slowly.

People who look forward to a happy marriage and a fulfilling sex life take good care of their bodies. They avoid any practice that might impair their physical, emotional, and spiritual life.

Singleness

In sharing these ideas about sex with you, I have assumed that practically all of you, in the normal course of events, will marry. This does not take into account wars, nuclear holocausts, or the long-wished-for coming of Jesus.

Something should be said at this point about the condition of singleness. Some persons never marry. As Christians they lead lives of chastity. They are able to direct sexual energy into other avenues of activity and in ways that produce enriched and productive lives. Maintaining such a life of singleness requires a steady control over the sex drive.

Single women, generally, find themselves in that condition because they have not had offers of marriage or have had the good sense to turn down some proposals that would have led to unhappy marriages and poor parenthood. Others may avoid marriage because of an abnormality in sexual orientation, a basic immaturity, or a selfish refusal to accept the responsibility of building a marriage and a family.

Singleness also follows divorce or death. The great majority of people in these circumstances remarry. The period of singleness, however, can bring on a vulnerability to offers of sex. After years of marriage, sex can become part of the rhythm of life and can turn into a hunger that seeks satisfaction. Sex is often engaged in as a way to alleviate loneliness—the physical closeness is often misread as emotional closeness. Perhaps something should be written for these individuals.

I write this to be fair to single people, especially the women. They should never become the object of such "snide" remarks as "unclaimed treasure" or the out-of-date term "old maid."

So keep a sensible balance on this subject as you move on in years (and in wisdom).

Chapter 11

Looking Ahead to Marriage— What E. G. White Says

Almost all of you are looking forward to marriage in the not-too-distant future (all plans subject, of course, to "God willing"). You should, for your own good and happiness, read *Messages to Young People* and *The Adventist Home*.

I recognize that most young people don't heed such advice. Perhaps reading those two books seems like an overwhelming task. But I would guess that even a slow reader could get through both books in ten or twelve hours. You can spread the reading time over a period of three to four months and let the God-given advice sink in like a slow, gentle rain. That way you can go through periods of growth between sittings.

Believe me when I say that reading and applying Mrs. White's counsel will save you a lot of grief and regret. Following her suggestions comes the closest to a guarantee that you can find for a permanent and totally satisfying marriage. And surely you wish for all the good things that can last through the years—as you become "old" like your parents. (Again, I recognize the strong possibility that the Lord may return very soon.)

If you haven't already read these fine books, let me have the privilege of sharing with you some of the material they contain. I am arranging the quotations by subject, though you will quickly notice that some of them overlap.

What Marriage Often Is Today

"Few have correct views of the marriage relation. Many seem to think that it is the attainment of perfect bliss. . . . Marriage, in a majority of cases, is a most galling yoke. There are thousands

121

that are mated but not matched" (AH 44).

"The majority of the marriages of our time and the way in which they are conducted make them one of the signs of the last days" (AH 71).

"The marriage institution was designed of Heaven to be a blessing to man; but, in a general sense, it has been abused in such a manner as to make it a dreadful curse. Most men and women have acted in entering the marriage relation as though the only question for them to settle was whether they loved each other" (MYP 461).

"Satan is constantly busy to hurry inexperienced youth into a marriage alliance. But the less we glory in the marriages which are now taking place, the better" (MYP 455).

Important Things to Consider in Planning Marriage

Use Judgment, Accept Counsel—"If there is any subject that should be considered with calm reason and unimpassioned judgment, it is the subject of marriage" (AH 70).

"I have the most painful sense of helplessness when parties come to me for counsel upon this subject. I may speak to them the words that God would have me; but they frequently question every point, and plead the wisdom of carrying out their own purposes; and eventually they do so.

Advice is only thrown away on those who are determined to have their own way. Passion carries such individuals over every barrier that reason and judgment can interpose" (MYP 458, 459).

Listening to Parents—"Wise parents will never select companions for their children without respect to their wishes" (AH 75).

"A young man who enjoys the society and wins the friendship of a young lady unbeknown to her parents does not act a noble Christian part toward her or toward her parents" (AH 57).

Weighing Effects of Marriage on Both of You—"Let the questions be raised, Will this union help me heavenward? Will it increase my love for God? And will it enlarge my sphere of usefulness in this life?" (AH 45).

"No one can so effectually ruin a woman's happiness and usefulness, and make life a heartsickening burden, as her own husband; and no one can do one hundredth part as much to chill the hopes and aspirations of a man, to paralyze his energies and ruin his influence and prospects, as his own wife. It is from the marriage hour that many men and women date their success or failure in this life, and their hopes of the future life" (AH 43).

Engaging in Prayer—"Jesus has purchased you with His own life; you belong to Him; therefore He is to be consulted in all things, as to how the powers of your mind and the affections of your heart shall be employed" (AH 54).

"If men and women are in the habit of praying twice a day before they contemplate marriage, they should pray four times a day when such a step is anticipated. . . . A sincere Christian will not advance his plans in this direction without the knowledge that God approves his course" (MYP 460).

"Those professing to be Christians should not enter the marriage relation until the matter has been carefully and prayerfully considered from an elevated standpoint, to see if God can be glorified by the union." (MYP 462).

Characteristics to Watch For—(In men) "Is his life pure? Is the love which he expresses of a noble, elevated character, or is it a mere emotional fondness? . . . Will she be allowed to preserve her individuality? . . . Has . . . [her] lover a mother? What is the stamp of her character?" (AH 47).

(In men) "Under such guidance [of God-fearing parents, and Christ through the Bible and prayer] let a young woman accept as a life companion only one who possesses pure, manly traits of character, one who is diligent, aspiring, and honest, one who loves and fears God" (MYP 435).

(In men) "Listen not to the proposals of a man who has no realization of his responsibility to God" (AH 48).

(In women) "Let a young man seek one to stand by his side who is fitted to bear her share of life's burdens, one whose influence will ennoble and refine him, and who will make him happy in her love" (MYP 435, 436).

(In women) "Will she be one who will be patient and painstaking? Or will she cease to care for your mother and father at the very time when they need a strong son to lean upon? And will she withdraw him from their society to carry out her plans and to suit her own pleasure, and leave the father and mother who, instead of gaining an affectionate daughter, will have lost a son?'' (AH 46).

Understanding What Love Is and Is Not—''There is but little real, genuine, devoted, pure love. This precious article is very rare. Passion is termed love'' (AH 50).

''True love is a high and holy principle'' (AH 50).

''True love is not a strong, fiery, impetuous passion. On the contrary, it is calm and deep in its nature. It looks beyond mere externals, and is attracted by qualities alone. It is wise and discriminating, and its devotion is real and abiding'' (AH 51).

''Imagination, lovesick sentimentalism, should be guarded against as would be the leprosy'' (AH 51).

''That love which has no better foundation than mere sensual gratification will be headstrong, blind, and uncontrollable'' (AH 51).

''Like some epidemic, or contagion, that must run its course, is the infatuation that possesses them [a couple]; and there seems to be no such thing as putting a stop to it'' (MYP 456, 457).

Courtship Feelings and Conduct Displeasing to God

''The iniquity that is cherished by young as well as old . . . [and] the unwise, unsanctified courtship and marriages cannot fail to result in bickerings, in strife, in alienations, in indulgence of unbridled passions, in unfaithfulness of husbands and wives, unwillingness to restrain the self-willed, inordinate desires, and in indifference to the things of eternal interest'' (AH 53).

''You have fallen into the sad error which is so prevalent in this degenerate age, especially with women. You are too fond of the other sex. . . . You encourage, or permit a familiarity which does not always accord with the exhortation of the apostle, to 'abstain from all appearance of evil.' . . .

''Turn your mind away from romantic projects. You mingle with your religion a romantic, lovesick sentimentalism, which does not elevate, but only lowers'' (AH 52).

''The young are bewitched with the mania for courtship and marriage. Lovesick sentimentalism prevails'' (AH 52).

''The youth trust altogether too much to impulse. They should not give themselves away too easily, nor be captivated too readily by the winning exterior of the lover. Courtship as carried on in this age is a scheme of deception and hypocrisy, with which the enemy of souls has far more to do than the Lord" (AH 55).

"If there is any subject that should be considered with calm reason and unimpassioned judgment, it is the subject of marriage. If ever the Bible is needed as a counselor, it is before taking a step that binds persons together for life. But the prevailing sentiment is that in this matter the feelings are to be the guide; and in too many cases love-sick sentimentalism takes the helm and guides to certain ruin. It is here that the youth show less intelligence than on any other subject; it is here that they refuse to be reasoned with. The question of marriage seems to have a bewitching power over them. They do not submit themselves to God. Their senses are enchained, and they move forward in secretiveness, as if fearful that their plans would be interfered with by some one.

"The underhand way in which courtships and marriages are carried on is the cause of a great amount of misery. . . . On this rock thousands have made shipwreck of their souls. Professed Christians, whose lives are marked with integrity, and who seem sensible upon every other subject, make fearful mistakes here. They manifest a set, determined will that reason cannot change. They become so fascinated with human feelings and impulses that they have no desire to search the Bible and come into close relationship with God" (MYP 447, 478).

"Satan is busily engaged in influencing those who are wholly unsuited to each other to unite their interests. He exults in this work, for by it he can produce more misery and hopeless woe to the human family than by exercising his skill in any other direction" (MYP 455).

"Satan's angels are keeping watch with those who devote a large share of the night to courting. . . . The laws of health and modesty are violated. It would be more appropriate to let some of the hours of courtship before marriage run through the married life. But as a general thing, marriage ends all the devotion manifested during the days of courtship!

"These hours of midnight dissipation, in this age of depravity, frequently lead to the ruin of both parties thus engaged. . . . The good name of honor is sacrificed under the spell of this infatuation, and the marriage of such persons cannot be solemnized under the approval of God. They are married because passion moved them, and when the novelty of the affair is over, they will begin to realize what they have done. In six months after the vows are spoken, their sentiments toward each other have undergone a change. . . . The promises at the altar do not bind them together. In consequence of hasty marriages, even among the professed people of God, there are separations, divorces, and great confusion in the church" (MYP 457, 458).

"You must not imperil your souls by sowing wild oats" (AH 59).

" 'Thou shalt not steal' was written by the finger of God upon the tables of stone, yet how much underhand stealing of affections is practiced and excused!" (AH 58).

"The thought of marriage seems to have a bewitching power upon the minds of many of the youth. Two persons become acquainted; they are infatuated with each other, and their whole attention is absorbed. Reason is blinded, and judgment is overthrown" (MYP 456).

"If, in your infatuation, you can repeatedly turn from the prayer meeting, where God meets with His people, in order to enjoy the society of one who has no love for God, and who sees no attractions in the religious life, how can you expect God to prosper such a union? . . .

"The habit of frequently being in the society of the one of your choice, and that, too, at the sacrifice of religious privileges and of your hours of prayer, is dangerous; you sustain a loss that you cannot afford" (MYP 437, 438).

Immature Marriages

"Early marriages are not to be encouraged. A relation so important as marriage and so far-reaching in its results should not be entered upon hastily, without sufficient preparation, and before the mental and physical powers are well developed" (MYP 438).

Marriage With Unbelievers

"There is in the Christian world an astonishing, alarming

indifference to the teaching of God's word in regard to the marriage of Christians with unbelievers. Many who profess to love and fear God choose to follow the bent of their own minds rather than take counsel of Infinite Wisdom" (AH 61).

"Although the better judgment of the believer may suggest the impropriety of a union for life with an unbeliever, yet, in nine cases out of ten, inclination triumphs" (AH 65).

"My sister, unless you would have a home where the shadows are never lifted, do not unite yourself with one who is an enemy of God" (AH 67).

Recommended Behavior

"Let every step toward a marriage alliance be characterized by modesty, simplicity, sincerity, and an earnest purpose to please and honor God. Marriage affects the afterlife both in this world and in the world to come" (MYP 435).

"In all the deportment of one who possesses true love, the grace of God will be shown. Modesty, simplicity, sincerity, morality, and religion will characterize every step toward an alliance in marriage. Those who are thus controlled will not be absorbed in each other's society, at a loss of interest in the prayer meeting and the religious service" (MYP 459-460).

"Let woman give herself to Christ before giving herself to any earthly friend, and enter into no relation which shall conflict with this" (MYP 440).

Postscript

Dear Reader:

Well, I've finally come to the end. I have enjoyed sharing some of my ideas with you on sex. Perhaps you have found some that were helpful and many that reinforced those ideals you already have established.

I'd like very much to meet you in person. Since this is not possible, here's my parting wish for you:

"The Lord bless you and watch over you;
the Lord make his face to shine upon you
and be gracious unto you;
the Lord look kindly on you and give you peace."
—Numbers 6:24-26, NEB*

*From *The New English Bible.* © The Delegates of the Oxford University Press and the Syndics of the Cambridge University Press 1961, 1970. Reprinted by permission.